THE GUT MAKEOVER
RECIPE BOOK

JEANNETTE HYDE
Nutritional Therapist BSc.

Quercus

To Markus, Hanna and Max

First published in Great Britain in 2016 by

Quercus Editions Ltd
Carmelite House
50 Victoria Embankment
London EC4Y 0DZ

An Hachette UK company

A CIP catalogue record for this book is available
from the British Library.

PB ISBN 978 1 78648 152 8
EBOOK ISBN 978 1 78648 153 5

10 9 8 7 6 5 4 3 2 1

Typeset by e-type, Liverpool

Printed and bound in Great Britain by Clays Ltd, St Ives plc

Contents

Introduction

Dear Reader,

My first book, *The Gut Makeover*, explains how to help your gut bacteria make you healthy by eating 100 per cent real food for one month. It's this simple: leave out the junk and load up on delicious, unprocessed food to feed the beneficial bacteria in your digestive system. This will reduce your weight and digestive symptoms, and improve your mood, energy, sleep and skin health.

The Gut Makeover is an eating strategy for people who love food and want to feel great without tiresome calorie counting or going hungry. This practical book opens the door to delicious eating for one month, introducing you to strategies that you can build into your life in the longer term, so the benefits keep coming.

Thousands of readers are already reaping the benefits of *The Gut Makeover* and now this recipe book makes the lifestyle easier than ever. I'll help you conjure up quick, easy, delicious meals to nourish your microbes and give you beautiful skin, bags of energy and restful sleep – all that AND you'll see the pounds melt off.

What are the main principles of *The Gut Makeover* method?

You'll eat three hearty meals a day, avoid snacking, and do an easy and manageable 12-hour overnight fast. You'll include seven plants a day (five vegetables, two fruit), including lots of variety, colour and texture. You'll be encouraged to sprinkle fresh herbs, pomegranate seeds and spring onions and other colour onto your food at every opportunity. You'll eat good-quality protein cooked in extra virgin olive oil to keep you feeling full. This oil contains polyphenols (a particular type of plant chemicals) which the beneficial bacteria love to dine out on, and which protect the oil against damage at high temperatures.

In just a few weeks this way of eating will help you build a microbiome full of diversity and balance, with the beneficial bacteria in the majority and the pathogenic ones in the minority. Study after study has shown that you can manipulate your microbiome by feeding it simple, real food. Unprocessed food really is your medicine and this book contains more than 100 recipes designed to nourish your gut bacteria and help you feel and look great.

What are the main benefits and why?

Without doubt, the most talked-about result of *The Gut Makeover* is the weight loss – with most readers losing about half a stone (3.5 kilos) in a month, though some people have lost much more, or slightly less. This is without counting calories and without going hungry. When our gut bacteria are diverse and in balance, vexing digestive issues tend to subside and, interestingly, mood and anxiety often improve, too. The psychology department at St Mary's University Twickenham, in London, is currently conducting research on gut and mood symptoms before and after following *The Gut Makeover* for a month. When lead researcher Dr Kate Lawrence saw the first set of results she said the improvements in digestive and mood scores were dramatic: 'If these were the results of a drug, it would be front-page news,' she said. It is exciting work.

So it's good to hear that gut and mood symptoms can improve by feeding our gut bacteria the right stuff, but why does the weight melt away? When the bacteria are in balance they send signals to our hunger hormones telling us when we are full, and when we are hungry at the right points, so this helps control our weight and avoid overeating. This bacteria also influences calorie extraction from the food we are eating. When it is in balance, there is less aggressive caloric extraction from the food we are eating. Revolutionary. That is why there is no calorie counting on this plan.

This isn't a traditional 'diet' in the usual sense of the word – which so often spells deprivation, hunger and, for many people, failure. *The Gut Makeover* is an eating strategy, or a plan. You are taking your health in your own hands. Weight reduction is just one part of the benefits spanning your whole quality of life, from increased energy, better sleep, disappeared bloating, constipation, heartburn, IBS, eczema, acne, swollen ankles, headaches, itchy eyes, stuffy nose, sneezing attacks, chronic coughing and dry skin.

Why I've written this book

Like many women, I've struggled with my weight, energy levels and mental health over the years. Over a decade ago I had a challenging and busy job as a journalist in a newspaper office, while juggling a young family, then I burnt out. I felt as if there wasn't time to take care of myself and after the crash, when I was looking for answers to my health, I was confused. The only 'solution' offered to me by my GP was to take anti-depressants, which made me feel even more lousy. These drugs were offered after seeing several specialists who all told me they couldn't reach a diagnosis (physically I couldn't move my neck for several months, as well as feeling low)! I used to read magazine and newspaper articles about nutrition, but everywhere I looked for answers seemed to suggest a different and conflicting approach. I wanted to be able to evaluate research papers and design a diet for myself based on cutting-edge research that works. I took the most thorough route available to becoming a nutritional therapist by doing a four-year BSc honours degree at Westminster University. This book is a culmination of evaluating latest research, what I have learnt from working with hundreds of clients on their diet as a nutritional therapist, and being a working mother who needs to be able to produce nourishing meals for a family in little time.

Plan, plan, plan!

As a working mum myself, I know how important it is that *The Gut Makeover* fits around a busy family life. It may involve a bit more planning than you may be used to, but once you are up and running it becomes habit. Almost every meal you make, I encourage you to make extra so that you have delicious leftovers the next day. Many of the recipes are also family friendly and easy to knock up after work, and almost all of the ingredients used are available in high-street supermarkets. I've also shared my experience of how to make your own fermented milk kefir (cow's, goat's or coconut varieties if you are dairy intolerant) in response to numerous emails and online requests. Once you get into the habit of nourishing your gut, thinking colour and fibre will become second nature, but making fermented food may also become an enjoyable and satisfying sideline – it certainly has been for me and many others. I've also included some more unusual recipes, too, so you can even do a *Gut Makeover* dinner party and no one will know they are being *Gut Makeovered*!

And finally...

The Gut Makeover is not about deprivation; it's about abundance. Just eat real food for one month. Real food is more powerful than any drug or any supplement. Take your health into your own hands, your own cooking hands. Try it – you will be astonished at the results.

How to use this book

This book centres around a four-week plan that I have designed based on the latest research on the microbiome and impaired intestinal permeability (also known as leaky gut, see page 16). *The Gut Makeover* is not a diet in the popular sense of the word; it is a restoration programme. It's a whole-health overhaul.

For four weeks we are going to take out of your everyday diet the foods which could be irritating your gut lining or skewing the balance and impacting the diversity of that 1.5kg of bacteria in your intestines, and replace them with foods which will help. Think of it as a personal makeover working from the inside out; using good food to restore your bacteria, to create a knock-on impact on your weight, skin, mood and immune system.

The four-week plan pays a nod to the diets of the indigenous hunter-gatherers of South America and Africa who have wide species of bacteria in their guts that are supported by eating many vegetables, and supplemented with quality meats and fish, eggs, nuts and seeds and, from time to time, a little dairy. The plan involves eating a diverse array of delicious, unprocessed foods which won't leave you hungry.

Once we have built up your gut to a state of bacterial diversity and abundance on the four-week makeover, we will transition to the maintenance part of this programme, which is a gut-friendly version of the real Mediterranean diet, based on the diet from the pre-1960s in Greece. This consisted of a high intake of plants – vegetables, seasonal fruits and wild herbs – supplemented with fish, nuts and grains, virgin olive oil, artisan slow-matured cheeses teeming with friendly bacteria, and moderate amounts of quality meat. This Mediterranean diet is the best way to support a healthy gut. It's also an enjoyable way to eat for the long term.

By following this plan you will implement a set of habits that you can incorporate into your diet every day. Once you have a strong gut lining and a flourishing, healthy pond of beneficial bacteria, you will go forward with a set of principles to keep it that way. The recommendations in these pages are simple and implementable, so you can attain and maintain a tip-top-condition gut and enjoy good health and weight even after the four weeks are up. You may, from time to time, come back to the four-week plan. It isn't a rollercoaster of feast and famine, self-denial and rebound hunger, it's simply a hit of the reset button.

To help make the diet easy, lists of recommended natural and unprocessed foods are included as a starting point for the four-week plan. Use the ingredients on pages 42-50 to create some of your own meals or make a few simple adaptions to any favourite recipes you already have. Real-life case studies are included throughout this section to give a taste of the challenges and successes that other dieters experienced during their own four-week journey as well as a list of frequently asked questions to cover any eventuality.

An entire chapter of delicious recipes follow to keep you inspired throughout the plan and beyond. There are ideas for breakfast, lunch and dinner as well as sensible food substitutions and plenty of sample meal plans to see you through the four-week phase. Useful advice on what to eat if you're dining out will help you to avoid the common pitfalls that might tempt you back into an unhealthy eating pattern.

A complete list of helpful websites and books for reference appears at the back of the book to support readers through the whole process and favourite ingredients are listed along with recommended suppliers and stockists to make food prep a cinch.

Why *The Gut Makeover* works

A road map of the gut

To put my ideas into context, let's have a quick tour of the digestive system. The tube that runs continuously from mouth to anus is a major highway that passes through the body. It is finally beginning to be acknowledged that much of our health is dependent on this highway performing optimally. A problem occurring near the beginning of the journey, such as at the mouth or stomach, can have a big impact on the gut lining and bacteria balance further down the highway. This effect becomes clearer when we can see what happens when it is operating well.

The mouth

The first stage of digestion happens in the mouth itself. This is where the mechanical breakdown of food occurs, as we grind and chew it with our teeth. Digestion is also aided by the release of enzymes; these are like chemical scissors, snipping food into smaller molecules so that they can be absorbed into our bloodstream further down the line. Some of these enzymes are released in our saliva.

The stomach

Once the food has been broken down by the teeth and mixed around with saliva, it goes down the chute (the oesophagus) to the stomach. The stomach is a dynamic organ, which can stretch in size to accommodate larger quantities of food. It produces hydrochloric acid and more enzymes, which work to further break down the arriving food, rather like a washing machine. The mashed-up food is then pumped through to the next chamber gradually. It usually takes about four to four and a half hours for a meal to leave the stomach.

The small intestine

When the food enters your small intestine it should now be sludge, known as 'chyme'. At this point, bile and more digestive enzymes join the chyme to help break it down into smaller and smaller particles. The food takes three to six hours to pass through this tube, and this is where the big, important action of absorption of fuel and nutrients into our bloodstream happens. The sludge is squeezed along and has quite a way to go. The texture of the inside of this long tube has the appearance of a shag-pile carpet: each strand is dotted with microvilli, which look like the bristles on a brush and are, unsurprisingly, known as the brush border. The shag pile and brush hairs have been designed to provide an enormous surface area for ease of absorption. The nutrients go through the little junctions between the blades of the brush border and shag piles into our bloodstream to fuel us, and the leftovers are transferred to the large intestine.

Our shag-pile carpet gets a huge amount of traffic every day, so it can wear out quickly, and if the junctions between the shags come loose or are torn – or if there is less mucus than normal – our absorption, and consequently our whole health, can be compromised.

The large intestine – and the microbiome

The large intestine is shorter and fatter than the small intestine, and this is where any water is absorbed. The residues – think of vegetables with particularly hard-to-break-down strands and material – provide food for the trillions of microbes. These leftovers spend up to two days in this department before they are excreted from the body.

In science, the colon used to be a forgotten and dismissed part of the digestive system, until the microbiome came along. Of course, this pond of bacteria had always been there, it just hadn't had much recognition before.

So what do these microbes do?

- They ferment indigestible fibres from plants such as vegetables to release short-chain fatty acids. The short-chain fatty acid from fibre that you will hear most about is called butyrate. This is a fuel that is needed to build the mucus which lines the gut. The mucus protects the gut lining, which is vital for a healthy immune system, mental health and good skin.
- They may determine how aggressively calories are extracted from the food we eat.
- They interact with our hormones – particularly the ones that tell us we are full or hungry.
- They manufacture B vitamins, which are needed for good mental health and to make us feel energised.
- They make vitamin K, which is needed to clot our blood if we have an accident, a cut or a graze.
- They interact with our immune cells.
- They interact with our nervous system.

Gut problems

So what does the digestive system look like when things go wrong? Here are the main potential problems:

IBS

Irritable bowel syndrome (IBS) is a catch-all term used by the medical profession to diagnose digestive problems where the cause is unknown. 'IBS' patients often have constipation, or loose stools, or alternate between the two. There is thought to be a stress and emotional component involved and sometimes this can indeed be the main underlying factor. However, in my clinical practice I've seen many times that what has been labelled 'IBS' is actually impaired intestinal permeability or dysbiosis. In my experience, removing the root cause of those (poor diet or foods that an individual may be intolerant to) and implementing a gut-friendly diet (*Gut Makeover* style) often leads to a vast improvement in IBS symptoms.

Dysbiosis

I've described the microbiome as a teeming pond of life, with different communities and species of bacteria living in it. When we eat a gut-friendly diet this pond will be in a happy balance. When this happens, it means the friendly bacteria ('commensal bacteria') are likely to be dominant and the unfriendly bacteria ('pathogens'), the lurgies, are kept in the background. If the lurgies become dominant, this is when we can run into health problems and possible 'dysbiosis'.

One of the first things a person with dysbiosis may notice is that their abdomen bloats and they experience more wind than usual. Others might find they start catching colds because their immune system is affected, or they might feel emotionally low. Recent research indicates that mood disorders can be connected with disharmony in the gut. Another consequence of dysbiosis is skin complaints, such as breaking out in spots or a worsening of eczema. Dysbiosis is also thought to result in greater numbers of calories being extracted from the food we eat.

Not chewing our food properly can also lead to undigested particles of food reaching the colon, where the non-beneficial bacteria feed on the undigested food (which isn't supposed to be there) and proliferate. Also, if the stomach doesn't produce as much acid as it should, the breakdown of food is compromised and the chance of undigested food reaching the colon and causing dysbiosis is increased. An indication of low stomach acid can be heartburn.

Low numbers of different species

Obese individuals have been shown to have a lower number of different species living in their guts than non-obese individuals. Eating a diet that incorporates a wide range of plants every day will create a wide diversity of different species of bacteria to flourish and call your colon home.

Leaky gut (impaired intestinal permeability)

In our tour of the digestive system I described the inside lining of the small intestine as being like a shag-pile carpet. When we're healthy (and chew our food properly) our food should break down to the lowest common denominator of particles and then travel through the shag-pile carpet, through minuscule gaps called tight junctions. However, sometimes these gaps can become wider, or ripped, and if this happens, undigested particles of food, or toxins, can seep through the shag pile into our bloodstream, which causes our immune system to go into a state of alarm.

These rips or gaps can occur for a number of reasons. Perhaps we haven't chewed well, or our stomach isn't producing enough stomach acid at the moment. It could be that we are stressed or drink a lot of alcohol. We may be continuing to eat foods that our body can no longer tolerate. Then there are the foods that haven't been broken down properly that can become potential irritants to the gut lining.

A healthy microbiome has been shown to help prevent leaky gut and reverse it. By following *The Gut Makeover* you will remove potential gut-lining irritants to give the villi and microvilli time to repair. Instead, you will eat foods that will help with the restoration of the gut-lining cells and beneficial bacteria in the colon.

Food intolerances

We can develop problems digesting certain food types when we are overexposed to them, particularly if we have a genetic predisposition to them (e.g. coeliac disease or non-coeliac gluten sensitivity, see box on page 23). This can cause an array of nasty symptoms, such as gas, bloating and indigestion. Food intolerances can also lead to other gut problems, such as leaky gut, which can in turn lead to dysbiosis.

A common problem food group is dairy. For example, it is estimated that 80 per cent of individuals of Asian heritage have difficulties digesting lactose, the natural sugar in milk. The genes of many cultures in Europe have adapted to tolerate dairy foods over the last 10,000 years, and lactase persistence (the production of the enzyme to break down lactose beyond infancy when it is needed to digest breast milk) has become common. In many Asian and African cultures, where dairy farming was less adopted, genes have not adapted so frequently to persistently produce lactase into adulthood.

The Gut Makeover removes common triggers of digestive discomfort such as gluten and all other grains for one month. Milk products are removed for the first fortnight then put back into the diet in prescriptive amounts in the second fortnight. At the end of the month, common allergens such as gluten and other grains are gradually reintroduced to help you identify if any particular ones are a problem for you personally. The aim of this approach is to create a tailormade diet that fits your particular physiology in the long term.

WHAT IS INFLAMMATION AND WHY SHOULD I CARE?

Acute inflammation can be a protective and helpful response in the body, but if the body keeps thinking it is injured, or that foreigners may be in its territory, this can trigger long-term inflammation that's detectable in your bloodstream, called 'systemic inflammation'. Your immune system could, for instance, start mounting an immune reaction every time you eat a food you might be sensitive to (such as gluten) or if undigested particles of food are entering the bloodstream because you have leaky gut. Dysbiosis can also lead to systemic inflammation. When the gut bacteria is in balance it is thought to promote anti-inflammatory signalling to the immune system.

Systemic inflammation has been linked with heart disease, and a mounting body of evidence indicates that inflammation is more dangerous than total cholesterol levels themselves. It is becoming apparent that what is much more dangerous than total cholesterol levels is if your arteries are inflamed – which means certain types of small particle-size cholesterol (as opposed to the fluffy, big type) stick to them.

The Western diet

In the last few decades we have lost many gut-supportive habits and foods. Traditional staples, such as slow-cooked stews and cheap cuts of meat – including organ meats – have become scarce, as have the habits of eating meat (or fish) and two veg, regularly eating greens, eating fish on Fridays, making chicken stock from leftover bones, drinking live yoghurts or fermented foods and eating slow-produced quality breads such as sourdoughs and smelly cheeses. Instead, a typical modern Western diet is based around convenience foods and packaged items.

Here are some of the food and drink items that are most commonly found in our diets:

1. **Refined carbohydrates** – such as white bread, pasta, rice and breakfast cereals. These are quickly broken down into sugar in the body.
2. **Sugar** – from white sugar in biscuits, cakes and breakfast cereals to high-fructose corn syrup in fizzy drinks. High-sugar diets have been linked with an impoverished microbiome.
3. **Trans fats** – these fats can be found in some commercial and highly processed cakes, biscuits, muffins, etc., and in some margarines and low-fat spreads. They can also be produced when oils are heated repeatedly to high temperatures with deep-frying. They come under names such as 'partially hydrogenated' fats and can sometimes be hard

to spot. Trans fats are the ones that cause most concern in connection to heart disease and brain function; they have been shown to raise inflammation markers, and, as mentioned on page 18, systemic inflammation has now been linked with heart disease and depression. We should look for quality and purity, selecting natural fats such as pure virgin olive oil, butter and coconut oil, as opposed to chemically manufactured fats such as those whose molecular structure changes to a trans fat during repeated deep-frying or chemical manufacture.

4. **Artificial sweeteners** – from aspartame to saccharin and sucralose. We think we are only consuming them when we have diet colas and fizzy drinks, but they are creeping into our other foods in the most unexpected places. Having heard that sugar is the spawn of the devil, we now head towards the 'reduced-sugar' ketchup, only to find it has been spiked with artificial sweeteners.

5. **Alcohol** – this has been shown to zap our gut flora and cause dysbiosis.

Here are some of the key areas where our Western diet is currently going wrong.

Low vegetable intake

The government advises us to eat five portions a day (a portion being about a cupful), however, myriad other sources indicate that we should be eating at least seven portions a day, if not more.

Lack of diversity

The more diverse your intake of plants and wider range of flora, the better your health and weight. If we want a beautiful microbiome we need to eat a rainbow of colours and a wide spectrum of varieties.

Too much sugar

A high-sugar diet can be detrimental to our microbiome. The reason for this is that bacteria love sugar, and the non-beneficial ones are likely to get more dense and powerful if we feed them sugar all day, leading to dysbiosis. However, if the rest of your digestion is working well, 85 per cent of sugar should have been absorbed before the food reaches the colon.

Too much caffeine

A digestive system constantly assaulted with caffeine from coffee, tea, colas, sports drinks and even green tea is unlikely to be operating at its best. Caffeine is a stimulant and can trigger the release of the stress hormones adrenaline and cortisol to get us going. When stress hormones are high, the sympathetic nervous system, known as the 'fight or flight' system, is dominating. This means the parasympathetic nervous system – 'the rest and digest' nervous system, which needs to be switched on to ensure our digestion is working well – may be operating at half mast while the body diverts energy to the more pressing stress situation.

Caffeine also can lead to sugar being tipped from the liver, where it is stored, into the bloodstream. So when you have that first coffee of the morning it doesn't just give you an adrenaline surge but a sugar rush, too.

Overexposure to antibiotics

When you take a course of antibiotics for an illness, it is also likely to kill friendly bacteria in your gut. You may be left with dysbiosis and a smaller diversity of species in there. Antibiotics have been shown to reduce the diversity of the bacteria in the gut in three to four days, with the impact lasting for up to four years after treatment if you're maintaining a typical Western diet.

In addition to any antibiotics we take, we may also be being subjected to residues of antibiotics on a low level by consuming farmed fish, meats and dairy, as farmers routinely give prophylactic antibiotics to their livestock.

I'm not saying never take antibiotics – they can, of course, be life-saving. I'm simply saying that there is a time and a place for them and you need to weigh up the pros and cons carefully. If you do need a course of antibiotics, *The Gut Makeover* is the perfect way to kick-start your microbiome afterwards.

GLUTEN – TO EAT OR NOT TO EAT?

Gluten is a protein found in certain grains, most commonly wheat. For many people, gluten isn't a problem.

Coeliac disease is a life-threatening autoimmune disorder which is triggered by eating gluten. A coeliac's immune system sees gluten as an invader. After fighting the gluten onslaught for a time, the immune system gives up, gets totally confused and can no longer recognise the difference between gluten and the cells of the small intestine itself. The immune cells then start attacking the gut cells and destroying them. This means the body can no longer absorb food properly and the person becomes ill.

You can develop and be diagnosed with coeliac disease at any stage of life. It is not something you are necessarily born with, though there may be a genetic predisposition.

Another point to consider is that it is not always the protein gluten that is causing reactivity. In some people it can be other proteins in the wheat kernel. There is also the possibility that gluten is irritating the gut lining from overexposure; having a pause from gluten for a while gives the gut time to heal and allows the gut flora to repopulate.

The Gut Makeover removes gluten from your diet for one month, even if you don't have a sensitivity. Here is the rationale: leaving it out in the short term will encourage you to replace it with many more vegetables in your diet, which will aid microbiome restoration. This in turn may lead to weight loss as you may extract fewer calories from the food you eat. At the end of the month you may wish to reintroduce gluten into your diet – eating foods like sourdough bread might be helpful for some. Don't turn to commercial gluten-free products as these are often highly processed and loaded with sugar. Instead, eat real, home-made foods.

The four-week *Gut Makeover*

The four-week plan basics

Before going into the plan in depth, it's good to get to grips with the basics. Here is an outline of the key principles that are involved in the one-month gut transformation.

Before you start!

Choose when to start

Before you embark on your *Gut Makeover*, schedule a month in your diary and cordon off a period of time you think would work well for you. This plan is designed so that you can follow it while continuing to go about your busy life. Preparation is key to success, and it is important to give yourself the best chance by choosing the optimum timeframe to work in.

Measure your weight

If one of your goals from *The Gut Makeover* is to lose weight, I suggest you weigh yourself about a week before you start the plan. You may also like to make a note of your waist measurement. Do this before you start reducing your caffeine, alcohol and sugar intake in the pre-plan week.

Try not to get on the scales again until halfway through the makeover and then again at the end of the four-week plan. It can be an unhelpful pressure. There are so many small day-to-day fluctuations and variables to consider – such as how much fluid you have been drinking, your hormone balance and how often you are having a stool movement. You will need a month on the plan for your beneficial gut flora to proliferate and influence your metabolism, and for inflammation to diminish, so allow these mechanisms to kick in.

Preparation week

Alcohol, caffeine, artificial sweeteners and sugar may all adversely impact your gut flora and the condition of your gut lining. We want to give your digestive system a break from these substances during *The Gut Makeover* so that your gut lining can mend and your flora repopulate.

However, going cold turkey – particularly from caffeine – can create tiredness and headaches, so, to make the plan easier, try to come off them slowly before the makeover month to minimise the impact. I recommend starting to gradually cut down on alcohol and caffeine as well as any diet drinks containing artificial sweeteners such as aspartame or sugar in the week before *The Gut Makeover*.

Do note that 'decaffeinated' teas and coffees usually still contain a small amount of caffeine, so they aren't suitable for the plan. However, you might choose to use them to help you slowly transition off these drinks and then replace them with healthier alternatives. Good old plain water is great – preferably filtered, as it's more environmentally friendly than bottled and you don't risk the problem of leached plastics in your drink.

A lot of the sugar we have each week comes from liquid – often without our realising it. The biggest culprits are often fresh fruit juices that we buy in the fridge section of the supermarket. However, a third of the carton is often sugar (natural fructose sugar). If you drink a glass of juice every day, try watering it down over a few days and then switching to a glass of water in the morning with a peeled orange instead or a chopped-up piece of fruit with the fibre still in it for your vitamins.

If you are a daily wine or beer drinker, switch to smaller glass sizes. If you're a white wine drinker you could dilute it with fizzy water to become a spritzer.

Cutting out alcohol can seem off-putting at first, especially if you usually have alcohol every day to wind down, or to cushion nerves at social functions when you are meeting new people. In terms of building a healthy gut lining and a wide range of bacteria so that you build your resilience for the future, pausing alcohol for 4 out of 52 weeks this year could be one of the best things you do for your overall health.

Aim by the end of this pre-week to have removed drinks containing alcohol, caffeine, sugar and artificial sweeteners from your diet altogether, so that you are ready to hit the ground running on day one of *The Gut Makeover*.

Keep an eye out for hidden sugars

Cutting out sugar and sweeteners might sound simple, but it's actually far more complex than just looking for the word 'sugar' on the packaging. You'll need to become literate in the many different names that sugar and sweeteners can come under. Once you're familiar with these terms, you may be surprised at how many of the products in your cupboards contain secret sugars.

Here are just some of the many names to look out for on labels representing sugar, or sugar substitutes to avoid

- HFCS (high-fructose corn syrup)
- Fructose
- Fruit juice concentrate
- Glucose
- Glucose syrup
- Galactose

- Granulated white sugar
- Brown sugar
- High-maltose corn syrup
- Maltodextrin
- Muscovado
- Rice syrup
- Hydrogenated starch hydrolysates
- Mannitol
- Maltitol
- Treacle
- Invert sugar
- Artificial sweeteners (e.g. sucralose, aspartame and saccharin)
- Xylitol
- Agave syrup
- Stevia
- Coconut sugar
- Sorbitol
- Erythritol
- Dextrose
- Sucrose

Sugars to use extremely sparingly in this plan and during maintenance

- **Honey:** This is a natural prebiotic substance that will feed the beneficial bacteria in the gut. Honey is sweeter than sugar, so you need very little. It is a good option to include in your cooking in small treat portions. If you can afford it, choose raw honey, which has undergone less processing than regular honey so contains more enzymes, which are better for your digestion.

- **Maple syrup:** This is digested quickly so should only be used sparingly. It contains trace minerals such as manganese (which is needed to make energy in the body) and zinc (which is good for the skin). Make sure you use an unadulterated pure form (i.e. not one mixed with corn syrup).

What you can and can't eat on the plan

Alcohol: It is well documented in gut research that alcohol can damage the mucus in our small intestine and colon and can cause dysbiosis and leaky gut. Have you ever noticed your eczema is worse after a night out drinking? This could be a leaky gut. Or do you suffer loose stools as well as a poor mood the morning after a few drinks? That could be dysbiosis.

Caffeine: This a stimulant, which can lead to raised stress hormones and sugar levels in the blood. Lots of caffeine can also lead to the 'rest and digest' part of our nervous system potentially underperforming. *The Gut Makeover* avoids caffeine for one month to help improve your digestive system.

Sugar and artificial sweeteners: Both sugar and artificial sweeteners such as aspartame, saccharin and sucralose have been linked with suboptimal microbiomes, so for good gut health these are avoided this month.

Dairy (such as milk and cheese): Although included, dairy is limited in *The Gut Makeover*. This is because some individuals may have problems digesting it. However, in the 'reinoculate' part of the plan (weeks three and four) it is included in portion-controlled amounts because bacteria in foods such as fermented milk kefir can boost beneficial gut flora, helping weight control, mood balance and the immune system. For those of you who suspect you have or have had lactose intolerance diagnosed (usually through a breath test), we will suggest some gut-supporting non-dairy fermented foods.

Grains: Gluten-containing grains such as wheat, rye and spelt, etc., are not included in *The Gut Makeover* because they can irritate the gut lining in sensitive individuals. On *The Gut Makeover* you not only leave out the gluten-containing grains, but also all other grains, such as rice, oats and quinoa, so that you can fill their place on the plate with large portions of deliciously prepared vegetables. Grains can then be added back into your diet in the maintenance part of the programme, if you like.

Beans and pulses: These contain high levels of lectins, which when eaten in high quantities can cause leaky gut, bloating and dysbiosis in some individuals. However, pulses do contain prebiotic fibres, which can be beneficial to your gut flora in the long run. I have suggested vegetarians add them back into the diet at the end of the first fortnight, earlier than meat eaters, in order to have more choice of proteins to eat.

Nightshade vegetables: Potatoes, tomatoes, aubergines, peppers and chillies are all included in the plan. Some people choose to omit nightshade vegetables from their diet because, like pulses, they are higher in lectin proteins than a lot of other vegetables, but it is rare to find people who genuinely have a problem with them. I recommend including them, so the vitamins, minerals and wide array of plant chemicals in them can be exploited.

Fruit: Two pieces (or two cups) of fresh fruit are included in the makeover each day. Portion control will keep your sugar intake low while you still receive the benefits of the fibre, natural plant chemicals and nutrients in them. Dried fruit is excluded from the diet due to the copious amounts of fructose sugar in it – much more than when fruit is eaten fresh.

Weeks one and two: REPAIR

You've cut out the bad stuff in the preparation week – the hard bit is over – now it's time to start putting the good stuff into your diet.

Rethink your plate

On the most basic level, look at your plate – it should, ideally, be two-thirds plants, one-third protein.

Eat a large quantity and variety of plants

Crowd out the gluten and other grains, plus sugar, in your diet with tonnes of plant matter. Aim to eat at least seven (raw weight when chopped) cupfuls of plants per day instead: five as vegetables, two as fruit.

Alternatively, make a fist with your hand and imagine seven vegetables and fruit to the volume of seven fists.

For a diverse microbiome for good health, you need a varied diet. Aim to eat between 20 and 30 different varieties of vegetables (including herbs) and some fruits per week.

Improve your digestion with bitter leaves and other foods

Chewing bitter leaves such as rocket, chicory or radicchio trigger stomach-acid release, aiding digestion further. Get into the habit of having some bitter leaves and a vinai-grette dressing whenever you can – either as a starter, a side salad or even beefed up into a main meal. Your digestion may be improved, and you'll also clock up extra vegetable portions to benefit your gut, weight and health.

Sharp citrus fruits, such as lemon or grapefruit juice, are also triggers of stomach-acid production. Another trick is to eat fresh (not cooked) pineapple or papaya with your starters or main meals as they contain natural plant enzymes, a kind of chemical scissors, which help break down and make your overall meal easier to digest.

Include good-quality protein

To repair your gut lining throughout the four weeks, **eat protein from animals from the best sources you can access and afford.** The antibiotic load should be less from animals that have been reared organically. Less antibiotics in them means less antibiotic residues in you. This in turn should mean a healthier microbiome (as antibiotics kill gut flora) and less fat storage and weight gain.

For gut repair, **incorporate organ meats into your diet once or twice a week.** Meats such as chicken livers, ox hearts and kidneys are inexpensive nutrient powerhouses that build healthy gut linings. If you are vegetarian or don't like organ meats, you can get the vitamin A needed for building your gut lining from the yolk in eggs.

VEGETARIANS AND PROTEIN

In the first fortnight of the plan vegetarian sources of protein are eggs, nuts and seeds – up to 45–56g of protein a day.

Try to vary your selection of nuts and seeds as much as possible to broaden the range of types of proteins you eat

In the second half of the makeover, vegetarians can introduce pulses such as lentils and beans, so that there are more protein options to choose from.

You can quickly check the protein content (as well as other nutrients) of many foods here:

http://nutritiondata.self.com

Choose non-dairy fats in the first fortnight

Use non-dairy fats, such as virgin olive oil, to cook and make dressings as they contain particular plant chemicals called polyphenols, which have been linked with boosting bacteria in the gut. They also have anti-inflammatory properties and taste delicious. Coconut oil is also an option for cooking and is an anti-inflammatory. For more on using fats and oils during the plan, see pages 43–4.

Chew properly and relax

Move away from your desk and computer screen and switch off your phone when eating. **Try to chew each mouthful 20 times to stimulate the production of stomach acid and enzymes** to help digestion and absorption of your food, and to avoid dysbiosis in the colon. Chewing may also ease digestive complaints such as heartburn, burping, stomach pains, abdominal bloating, constipation or loose stools, as well as embarrassing wind.

Another big reason why chewing properly helps us to manage our weight is because we can identify when we feel full and so are less likely to overeat. It takes about 20 minutes for our satiety hormones to kick in after eating.

Replace quick cooking methods, with slow – or at least slow-style – ones . . .

Include stewed meats and casseroles in your cooking often. Meat that has been well cooked is easier to digest and to absorb nutrients from. There is less work for your stomach acid and those natural scissor cutters, your digestive enzymes, to do. Your gut flora won't be bombarded with undigested food, which could cause bloating, gas and possibly weight gain.

Fast overnight

Aim for a 12-hour overnight fast between dinner and breakfast. If you eat breakfast regularly at 7am, the last morsel of food passing your lips in the evening would be at 7pm. Or if you eat breakfast at 9am, don't eat anything after 9pm. This will help reset your microbiome, which in turn has a positive impact on your weight and health.

Weeks three and four: REINOCULATE

Congratulations! After two weeks you may have dropped a few pounds already. You may have more energy, established new habits and friends might be saying you look younger and your tummy is flatter.

It's time to put your foot on the gut bacteria accelerator for a bit more va va voom by eating fermented foods.

Step up 'prebiotic' vegetables and fruits

Prebiotic foods are those containing certain materials which cannot be broken down in the upper digestive system. When they reach the colon, they provide food for other bacteria. When these prebiotic fibres are combined with probiotic foods, they can boost your flora even more.

On page 49 you will find a list of prebiotic fruit and vegetables. It is best to build up your intake of prebiotic plants gradually in weeks three and four to avoid wind; start with half a banana, or a small banana each day, and go from there.

Prebiotic foods are attracting a lot of research attention and are being touted as potentially being even more important than probiotic fermented foods for their health benefits. The thinking is that you can boost your good bacteria in the gut by eating them and they are also good for weight loss because the fibre in them makes us feel fuller for longer. This is worth bearing in mind if you can't tolerate probiotic fermented dairy or miso foods.

COLD POTATOES

Cold potatoes may sound like an odd prebiotic, but once cooled after cooking they form a type of fibre in them called resistant starch. This starch can't be digested anywhere else except the colon. It can make you feel full up as it stays in the digestive system a long time, and can help with weight loss because resistant starch acts as a food for your bacteria. This is why only cold potatoes (such as in potato salads), rather than hot ones, are suggested throughout *The Gut Makeover*.

Introduce 'probiotic' foods to boost gut flora

Probiotic foods are those that contain live bacteria. In the first fortnight of the plan, dairy foods are left out of the diet to give your gut a chance to repair itself and avoid inflammation. However, during the reinoculation stage we can add back in some specific dairy products which contain live bacteria that have jobs to do.

A little fermented milk called kefir (see below) and also a small crumble of Roquefort cheese are good foods to introduce at this stage.

Not having had dairy for a fortnight by this time, it's good to take note of any digestive symptoms. If all is OK, have a bit more kefir the next day, or Roquefort. You could also use other types of fermented foods to boost your bacteria – sauerkraut or pickled fermented vegetables may do the trick.

Kefir fermented milk

Kefir and fermented milks are used in traditional cooking in many parts of the world. It is a staple of the diet in much of Eastern Europe (see page 196 for suppliers and stockists).

Kefir does not contain sugar (or artificial sweeteners) and its numbers of bacteria are usually into the double figures of billions. The more friendly bacteria in the kefir the better, and the more chance the stragglers have of getting through to your lower gut, where they can bloom away.

Kefir tastes a bit like fizzy milk! Whizz berries and other fruits into it for a delicious drink or add a banana containing prebiotic fibres, on which the probiotic bacteria from the kefir can have a feeding frenzy.

Roquefort cheese

This French cheese is particularly smelly and is fermented for a long time to create lots of bacteria, which your gut may love. It is delicious crumbled into salads or used as a topping.

Try to get the real Roquefort, not cheap copies, for its full impact. Do portion-control the cheese, though – a matchbox-size portion should be the maximum at one meal. If you cannot tolerate dairy, add live fermented miso to your cooking every day for the last two weeks of this plan.

Other foods to reintroduce or add

Butter (or organic ghee)

Butter tastes good and also comes with a fatty acid called butyrate, which helps build a healthy gut lining, so it can carry on some of the good work you have done in the first fortnight.

If you have problems digesting dairy, try using organic ghee. Ghee contains just 1 per cent lactose and minuscule traces of the protein casein, so many people who are lactose intolerant or can't digest casein can still often benefit from it without problems. Ghee also contains butyrate, to strengthen the gut lining.

Fermented tempeh

If you're vegetarian, this is a good protein addition at the halfway point of the plan.

In the *Gut Makeover*, usual supermarket highly processed tofus and processed soya foods are left out as they can irritate the gut lining. However, in Asia, fermented soya, such as tempeh, is thought to be key to better hormonal health for women. You can buy fermented tempeh in blocks from independent health-food stores and Asian supermarkets. You can add it to stir-fries and salads. A recipe is included on page 96.

What are you going to eat?

The following food lists are designed to fill the core of your shopping lists and to stock your store cupboard and freezer.

Foods listed in these categories are just a starting point; feel free to expand the range of quality protein and vegetables if you are more adventurous, or have better access to them. If you think of a meat, fish, seafood, egg or plant that is not here, do explore them if you fancy them. However, you should stick with the suggestions for probiotic foods and oils, as these are very specific to this programme. The key principle is to try to buy food as close to its original state as possible.

Meat, fish, seafood and eggs

Meat

- Beef
- Buffalo
- Chicken
- Duck
- Lamb
- Pork
- Turkey
- Organic chicken livers
- Organic calf's liver
- Kidneys
- Ox heart

Game

- Boar
- Grouse
- Pheasant
- Quail
- Rabbit
- Venison

Fish and shellfish

- Anchovies
- Cod
- Crab
- Haddock
- Herring
- Mackerel
- Mussels
- Oysters

- Prawns
- Salmon
- Sardines

- Scallops
- Trout
- Tuna

Eggs

From hens, ducks or quails.

Chicken stock

I've included a recipe for how to make real chicken stock on page 184, and I suggest you spoon it into your cooking – from soups and stews to stir-fries – at every opportunity for the collagen to support a strong gut lining.

Shy away from commercial chicken stock cubes if you can – they often contain artificial flavour enhancers and sometimes gluten – or highly processed forms of soya. Real chicken stock is now available in the fridge section of most supermarkets and is a better option.

Fats and oils

The fats and oils in this section have been chosen because they either contain substances shown to be good for the gut or have anti-inflammatory properties.

- Extra virgin olive oil or virgin olive oil (mechanical or cold pressed) – make these your main cooking oil and salad oils. Extra virgin olive oil comes from the first pressing of the olives so it has the highest content of plant chemical polyphenols useful for feeding your beneficial gut bacteria. Virgin olive oil comes from the second pressing. If you can afford extra virgin, that would be my top recommendation. Some readers have told me they spent the money they usually would spend on alcohol on extra virgin olive oil during this month

- Virgin coconut oil
- Real butter or ghee – in the second half of the month

Drinks

- Water – preferably filtered tap water
- Herbal teas, such as fresh ginger steeped in boiling water
- Unsweetened almond milk
- Coconut water
- Chicory root. This makes a good coffee replacement. It contains inulin, which is a prebiotic, to boost beneficial bacteria in the gut. It can be mixed with warmed unsweetened almond milk for a latte substitute, but take care to limit yourself to drinking one a day due to its potential laxative effect. Buy the 100 per cent organic chicory roasted powder if you can – beware of liquid versions, which are mixed with sugar

Nuts and seeds

These will be used principally in cooking. Nuts and seeds are highly nutritious and filled with minerals and vitamins. They also contain protein and fibre to fill you up, and the oils carry many health benefits, too. Many nuts contain zinc, which is necessary for a healthy gut lining.

Be careful on portions as high-fat diets have been linked with an unfavourable microbiome (as mentioned on page 20).

- Almonds
- Brazil nuts
- Cashew nuts
- Chestnuts
- Hazelnuts
- Macadamias
- Peanuts
- Pecans

- Pine nuts
- Pistachios
- Pumpkin seeds
- Sesame seeds (black or gold)
- Sunflower seeds
- Walnuts

Vegetables

Those marked in bold (overleaf) are prebiotic gut-flora boosters. You may need to introduce them slowly into your diet, as initially they can cause wind, but this should lessen as your gut flora becomes more balanced.

- **Asparagus**
- Aubergines
- Beetroot
- Broccoli
- Brussels sprouts
- Cabbage
- Carrots
- Cauliflower
- Celeriac
- Celery
- Chard
- **Chicory root**
- **Cold potatoes**
- Courgettes
- Cucumbers
- **Fennel**
- Green beans
- **Jerusalem artichokes**
- Kale
- **Leeks**
- Lettuce
- Mushrooms
- Okra (ladies' fingers)
- **Onions**
- **Pak choi**
- Parsnips
- Peas
- Peppers (capsicum)
- Pumpkin
- Radicchio
- Radishes
- Rocket
- Romanesco
- Salsify
- Spinach
- Squash
- Swede
- Sweetcorn
- Sweet potatoes
- Tomatoes
- Watercress

Herbs, spices and condiments

Many herbs are anti-inflammatory, as well as providing diversity for the microbiome and adding taste to your meals, so snip them up and use liberally.

- Basil
- Bay leaves
- Black pepper
- Cayenne pepper
- Coriander
- Cumin
- Dill
- Dried red chillies
- Fish sauce
- **Garlic**
- Ginger
- Kalamata olives
- Mint
- Mustard
- Pomegranate molasses
- Preserved or pickled lemons
- Rosemary
- Saffron
- Sea salt
- Sichuan peppers
- Sumac
- Tamari soy sauce
- Tarragon
- Thyme
- Turmeric (this is a powerful anti-inflammatory)
- Vinegars – including balsamic, red wine vinegar and apple cider vinegar

TIPS

- **Kalamata olives** are usually a purple colour. Do not eat the dark black olives which have been dyed – we want to keep your diet unprocessed.
- **Mustard** comes in a number of varieties. Go for French, not English, as English often contains gluten – though the powdered version doesn't.

- **Sea salt** contains minerals. I like Ibiza salt or Maldon.
- **Sichuan peppers (also known as Szechuan peppercorns or Sichuan flower chilli peppers)** are now stocked by some supermarkets, or you can get them online or from an Asian grocery store. They are worth the effort; they have a lovely lemony, peppery flavour.
- **Sumac** is popular in the Middle East and now available in supermarkets. It has a wonderful lime taste when rubbed into meats and fish.
- **Tamari sauce** is gluten-free, unlike soy sauce.
- **Vinegars** can be used in dressings or on salads.

Fruits

- **Apples**
- Apricots (*fresh* not dried)
- Avocados
- **Bananas**
- Blackberries
- Blackcurrants
- Blueberries
- Cherries
- Clementines
- Figs
- Gooseberries
- Grapefruits
- Grapes
- Kiwis
- Lemons
- Limes
- Mangoes
- Melons
- Mulberries
- Nectarines
- Oranges

- Papayas
- Passion fruits
- Peaches
- Pears
- Pineapples
- Plums
- Pomegranates
- Quinces
- Raspberries
- Rhubarb
- Satsumas
- Strawberries
- Tangerines
- Watermelons

Prebiotic foods

I've highlighted the prebiotic foods in the above lists using bold text, but here is a complete list of the approved prebiotic foods.

- Apples
- Asparagus
- Bananas
- Chicory root
- Cold potatoes (not hot!)
- Fennel
- Garlic
- Jerusalem artichokes
- Leeks
- Onions
- Pak choi
- Pulses (only allowed if you are vegetarian on the second half of the makeover to boost sources of protein)

Probiotic foods

- Kefir fermented milk – can be made from cow's, goat's or coconut milk. Coconut milk kefir can be a good option if you are intolerant to the proteins in animal milks. Some people who are intolerant to the sugar lactose in cow's or goat's milk are able to tolerate kefir made from the milk of these animals because much of the lactose has been broken down by the fermentation process. If you find you see a flare-up in your health condition when you have cow's milk kefir this may be because you are sensitive to the protein casein in it. In this case it may be worth trying goat's milk kefir, which does not contain casein, and has a different set of proteins in it which you may be OK with.

- Riazhenka (a Russian fermented drink made from baked milk)
- Roquefort
- Fermented live miso
- Fermented tempeh
- Sauerkraut
- Pickles such as gherkins – but read labels carefully as they must be properly fermented. The ones with high bacteria counts are usually sold in the fridge section of shops (see page 196 for recommended brands).

Strategies for success

If you don't normally cook from scratch, you may find this plan mildly challenging at first. However, once you're in a rhythm, have written your shopping lists, tried new recipes, packed your freezer, used your blender and perhaps started eating leftovers for lunch out of a plastic pot (not at your desk!), or found alternative items to sandwiches in the canteen or local lunch shops, habits will form and become part of your new routine.

The key to a successful *Gut Makeover* is the planning. If you go out unprepared, or without visualizing what the next meal will be, you may fall at the first hurdle. If it's late and you haven't got any *Gut Makeover* meals planned or defrosted, you may end up making poor food choices out of hunger and find yourself back where you started with your health.

At work, try to get into the habit of having fresh food with you in a box or just a piece of fruit, and warn colleagues that you are eating your own food when the ciabattas are trollied into meetings.

Have you thought about long-life foods you could have if stuck? Perhaps you could stash a jar of artichokes in olive oil, a tin of sardines, a tin or jar of olives, an apple and a bottle of coconut water in your desk drawer or car boot. I'm not suggesting this is the way to eat every day, but have your secret supports to help you keep on track.

If you know you struggle with willpower, think about asking a buddy to do *The Gut Makeover* with you. Doing it with your other half, flatmate, friend, colleague or neighbour can make the journey more fun, and can increase your chances of success as you can support each other along the way. On a practical level, you may even be able to save time by cooking in batches and swapping some of the portions with your buddy or neighbour without having to make two different meals. You can also swap recipes and ideas.

If you need more help to keep on track, join *The Gut Makeover* Facebook page. This online support group can be invaluable for sharing strategies and recipes and chatting to others with similar goals.

Eating Out à la Gut Makeover

Eating out is possible, but involves a little vigilance. All restaurants in the EU now have to provide lists of allergens in their foods by law, so finding out if something is *Gut Makeover*-friendly has never been easier, especially in chain restaurants which often have manuals behind the counter you can look at if you request one.

Many restaurants provide copies of their menus on their website, too. If I'm dining out with people who I don't feel comfortable quizzing the waiter/waitress in front of, I check out the menu online before I go, and ring ahead and chat through what I can eat. So when it comes to ordering, I know exactly what I'm going to have and the restaurant can easily provide, without any fuss or embarrassment. Yes, I know, I'm rather English like that!

Many restaurants will happily sauté a nice steak, or cook a piece of fish and produce a large salad or pile of crispy vegetables for you.

Indian

The Tandoori chicken or lamb are usually fine for the *Gut Makeover* and you shouldn't have to worry about sauce thickeners with gluten as these don't come with Tandoori dishes.

Indian restaurants are a great place to load up on vegetables that you don't normally cook yourself at home, so it's an opportunity to widen the variety you eat – try side dishes of ladies' fingers (okra), cauliflower, spinach, aubergines and tomatoes. Indian restaurants use plentifully the anti-inflammatories ginger and turmeric and, if you ask, can cook your meal in ghee (clarified butter), which contains butyrate for a healthy gut lining.

Japanese

The main challenge with Japanese restaurants is avoiding wheat, which is used in the making of regular soy sauce. Many restaurants use soy sauce as the main sauce, rather than tamari, which doesn't contain wheat, because it is cheaper. However, do ask for tamari. Many restaurants now offer it if you ask – Yo Sushi and Wagamama will both provide it on request. So, if you are looking for a meal in a sushi restaurant, go for a bowl of miso soup to start (avoid the bits of soya floating round unless the staff can confirm it is the fermented quality stuff, rather than the highly processed version). Then follow with a plate of sashimi fish slices with some sides of vegetables. Tuck into pickled vegetable sides. There are often plates of spicy marinated aubergines available; again, ask for yours to be made with tamari rather than regular soy sauce. Wagamama can adapt many of their dishes to a huge plate of plants with some protein – just ask – usually with lots of colour and variety. They do have a manual that staff can share with you explaining which dishes are wheat-/grain-/dairy-free, etc.

Italian and French

When ordering in Pizza Express, go straight to the main meal salad section and order a Niçoise salad; at Carluccio's, go to the meat and fish section and order from here avoiding gluten (they can often adapt), then order side dishes of vegetables or salads. In Café Rouge, order steak, roast chicken or grilled fish with vegetables or salad sides.

Portuguese

If in Nando's, order grilled chicken (check the marinade is gluten-free – it usually is, but check) and a couple of sides of vegetables, e.g. sweet potatoes (avoiding the dip), grilled sweetcorn, mixed leaf salad and peas in mint. Avoid, at all costs, the bottomless fizzy drinks!

Frequently asked questions

The Gut Makeover Facebook group (facebook.com/ gutmakeover) is our online community to get advice, ask questions and share tips and success stories. If you need more help to keep on track, press 'like' and follow updates and make contributions on *The Gut Makeover* Facebook page. This online support group can be invaluable for sharing strategies and recipes and chatting to others with similar goals, but I have included some of the most frequently asked questions here. Do come and join us online!

What should I do if I don't want to lose weight on *The Gut Makeover*, but I want to follow it for all the other health benefits that can come with it?

- Don't implement the 12-hour overnight fast.
- Have a mid-afternoon snack of nuts and fruit between lunch and dinner.
- Be more liberal with your oils and fats in cooking and include more fatty foods in the plan, such as nuts and seeds, avocados and coconut milk, and in the second fortnight be more generous with the Roquefort and the butter.

I've noticed after the first week I don't feel particularly hungry even several hours after breakfast.
Should I still try to eat protein with lunch, even if I
just fancy a vegetable soup or a light pile of salad?

In the first week of the plan it's important to have protein
with every meal as this anchors your blood sugar levels
and makes you feel full up for many hours. This means
higher chances of this plan being a success, as there is less
opportunity to fall into a state of ravenous hunger and
make poor food choices. If you don't feel hungry, adjust
your portion sizes to your reduced appetite.

What advice do you have for shopping and navigat-
ing the supermarket?

The shorter the ingredients list the better. If you don't
understand it, don't buy it. This plan is focused on
natural food. I like to look at ingredients lists on the sides
of food in supermarkets and think, 'If I was making that
myself would I put that in there?'

Are nuts and seeds counted in our 20–30 varieties
of plants each week?

Although, of course, these are plants, I suggest not
including them in the plant count so we can focus on the
bright colours and fibre that are filling your plate.

Is it OK to use frozen vegetables or fruit?

Yes! These foods contain lots of fibre and plant chemicals in their colour to feed beneficial bacteria, and are usually frozen soon after picking so retain many of their nutrients. Frozen peas, sweetcorn and berries are cheaper than fresh ones.

The 12 Principles

I hope that after *The Gut Makeover* you will look after your newly refurbished digestive system and enjoy the benefits. Here are 12 principles for maintaining a healthy gut lining and microbiome – and all the benefits that come with it – for the long term.

1. Implement a 12-hour fast habitually
2. Keep chewing, keep counting
3. Say adios to snacks
4. Keep up your seven a day
5. Go easy on pasta and grains
6. Invest in the least processed, most natural foods you can
7. Include fermented food and drinks daily
8. Use caffeine with caution
9. Use extra virgin olive oil as your default oil long term
10. Get dirty – dirt is good for the microbiome

11. Be cautious about antibiotic use
12. Ring-fence a few days a week when you don't drink, especially if you are a woman

The Mediterranean diet

So seven plants a day, as many different varieties and colours as possible, lots of fish, some meat – particularly wild or game, nuts and seeds, pulses (lentils, chickpeas, etc. – now your gut has repaired we can reintroduce these), sourdough bread (if you can tolerate it), extra virgin olive oil, a little red wine, a little dairy in the form of artisan-produced fermented cheeses from goats or sheep. Sounds good, doesn't it? And it would support a healthy digestive system very well, too.

That is essentially what the Mediterranean diet is, and it is easy to transition to after *The Gut Makeover*. If you follow the 12 principles above, your diet shouldn't be dissimilar to a real Med diet. Some of us may not want to keep a hunter-gatherer-style diet going forever, and with just a few tweaks could benefit and enjoy a Mediterranean-style diet for the long term.

Get Cooking! Recipes

Introduction

Now you've read the compelling science behind *The Gut Makeover*, here are the recipes for the four-week plan to transform your gut health. You'll be enjoying three deliciously varied meals a day, teeming with nutrients, without counting calories or going hungry.

Every meal includes mountains of vegetables and some fruits, cooked in delicious and enticing ways using the best of condiments, herbs and spices to keep life interesting and satisfying.

Note: Depending on their ingredients, some of these recipes are designed either for the first two weeks of the *Gut Makeover* ('Phase One'), or for the second two weeks ('Phase Two'). Others are suited for anytime in the month. All recipes are marked with a ①, a ② or both, to let you know which phase(s) they're best for.

Breakfasts

A liquid breakfast can be very easy and welcome in the morning – particularly when you're not terribly hungry.

Breakfast in a glass can slip down more easily than food you have to chew.

GREEN GUNGE ①②

Serves 2

I'm not going to mince my words – call a green smoothie what you like, but in the end it's basically gunge! It's palatable gunge, of course, and has the advantage of being a practical way to get lots of fibre and a variety of plants down you in one sitting. Here, the almonds are added for protein and good fats, which will keep you feeling full for longer. The ginger and mint are anti-inflammatory.

If you can't warm to the taste of a green smoothie but want to give it a go, sipping it through a straw will hide a lot of its flavour; but personally, with the zing of ginger and lime, I like this concoction.

2 cups kale or spinach, washed
1 cup filtered water
1 orange, peeled
50g almonds
3 fresh mint leaves
Juice of 1 lime
2cm fresh ginger, grated

Add all the ingredients to a blender and blitz.

Tip: If you have time, soaking the almonds overnight

in water makes it easier for your blender to break them up and easier for you to digest them.

PURPLE JUICE (is the new green juice) ①②
Serves 2

1 carrot, peeled
1 beetroot (you can use a cold ready-cooked or raw and
    peeled depending on how powerful your blender is!)
1 apple, peeled and cored
A handful of spinach leaves, washed
2cm fresh ginger, peeled and chopped
200ml filtered water

Add all the ingredients to a blender and pulse until smooth. Drink immediately, before the ingredients separate.

GREEN SHAKE ①②
Serves 2

2 handfuls of kale or spinach, washed
1 fennel bulb, chopped
2 ripe kiwi fruits
1 apple
¼ cucumber
1cm fresh ginger, unpeeled
½ lime, peeled
A handful of fresh mint leaves
250ml filtered water

Add all the ingredients to a blender and pulse until smooth. Taste for texture – if you prefer your shake a little less thick, add more water to dilute it. Drink immediately, before the ingredients separate.

NUTTY NON-DAIRY ① ②
BREAKFAST SHAKE

Serves 1

200ml unsweetened almond milk
½ cup frozen berries
½ banana
1 tbsp ground flaxseeds (also called linseeds)

Blend all the ingredients together in a blender until smooth and drink immediately. If left to stand, the shake will become thicker as the flax swells up, and then you'll need to eat it with a spoon.

Follow by drinking a glass of water to aid the digestion of the flaxseeds.

KEFIR and PINEAPPLE BREAKFAST SHAKE ②

Serves 1

If you are in a hurry you can use the ready-chopped pineapple that you find in the fridge section of the supermarket.

200ml organic kefir

1 cup chopped fresh pineapple

2cm fresh ginger, peeled

2 tsp chia seeds or ground flaxseeds

Add all the ingredients to a blender and pulse until smooth. Drink immediately, before the ingredients separate.

Follow by drinking a large glass of water to help the digestion of the chia or flaxseeds.

Tip: If you have time, soaking the chia seeds in water overnight makes it easier for your blender to break them up.

KEFIR and BERRIES ②

Serves 1

200ml organic kefir

1 cup frozen berries

½ banana

2 tsp chia seeds or ground flaxseeds

1cm fresh ginger, peeled and chopped

Blend all the ingredients together in a blender then drink immediately before the ingredients separate.

Tip: If you have time, soaking the chia seeds in water overnight makes it easier for your blender to break them up.

RED KEFIR SHAKE ②

Serves 1

Large handful of pomegranate seeds (you can buy fresh in
    the supermarket, ready extracted from the fruit)
200ml organic kefir
2cm fresh ginger, peeled and chopped
1 tbsp chia seeds

Add all the ingredients to a blender and pulse until smooth.
Drink immediately, before the ingredients separate.

    Follow by drinking a large glass of water to help the
digestion of the chia seeds.

PINK KEFIR SHAKE ②

Serves 1

Black cherries are rich in polyphenols to feed the good
bacteria in the gut. The kefir plants billions of good
bacteria in the gut, too. Ginger and chia or flax have
anti-inflammatory properties. For some people a shake
like this is filling enough in the morning, others may
need an egg, smoked salmon or a slice of banana bread
on the side to feel full until lunchtime. I recently found
these black cherries available year round frozen in
Tesco and I know Sainsbury's stock them too. As a

child I loved black cherry yoghurt in my packed lunches (which were probably full of sugar). This is a healthy and delicious alternative, and the flavour of the cherries is so good that you should not need to add any honey.

250ml organic kefir
A handful of black cherries (when out of season use straight from frozen)
2cm fresh ginger, peeled
1 tsp chia or flaxseeds

Add all the ingredients to a blender and pulse until smooth. Drink immediately, before the ingredients separate.

Follow by drinking a large glass of water to help the digestion of the chia seeds.

GRAPEFRUIT KEFIR ②

Serves 1

The tart flavours of this really wake you up in the morning. Nice followed by a couple of poached eggs for some protein and asparagus, so including the grapefruit you can tick off two plants before leaving the house. If you choose a pink grapefruit it gives the drink a pretty colour, but a yellow one would be fine too.

1 pink or yellow grapefruit
200ml organic kefir

Peel and take the seeds out of the grapefruit. Cut into pieces and place with the kefir in a blender and pulse until smooth.

POMEGRANATE ALMOND MILKSHAKE ①②

Chia seeds and flaxseeds both have anti-inflammatory omega-3 oils in them as well as protein and they help with digestion. I alternate the two in my breakfasts, to keep life interesting. If you're on a budget, opt for flaxseeds rather than chia, as they are usually much cheaper. The pomegranates here contain polyphenols to feed the beneficial bacteria in your gut. The ginger is anti-inflammatory.

There is a vast spectrum of almond milks on the market, some not very *Gut Makeover* friendly at all, containing gums and stabilisers. There are a few brands around with purer ingredients – literally just almonds, water and a little salt. See page 196 for suggested brands.

I find a shake isn't filling enough as a stand-alone breakfast for me. If you find that too, serve some protein on the side, such as an egg and smoked salmon, or a small omelette with a handful of spinach. That way you've clocked two of your seven a day (pomegranates and spinach) before even leaving the house!

80g pomegranate seeds
200ml unsweetened almond milk
2cm fresh ginger, peeled
1 tbsp chia or flaxseeds

Add all the ingredients to a blender and pulse until smooth. Drink immediately before the chia or flaxseeds expand, making the shake too thick to drink.

Follow by drinking a large glass of water to help digestion of the chia or flaxseeds.

RUSSIAN SHAKE ②

Serves 1

Riazhenka is a Russian cultured drink which is more creamy than kefir and tastes absolutely delicious. It is now available online and from many health-food stores. Like kefir, it usually lasts 2–4 weeks in the fridge, so can be bought in bulk and stored if ordering online.

250ml Riazhenka cultured baked milk drink
A handful of blueberries
1 tbsp chia seeds

Add all the ingredients to a blender and pulse until smooth. Drink immediately, before the ingredients separate.

Follow by drinking a large glass of water to help the digestion of the chia seeds.

GUT MAKEOVER BREAKFAST CEREAL ①②

(Phase 1)

Serves 1

A handful of blueberries

2 tbsp milled flaxseeds, almonds, Brazil nuts (you can buy
    mixes in packets from supermarkets, ready milled)

250ml unsweetened almond milk

1 tsp raw honey (optional)

Coconut water (optional)

Mix all the ingredients together in a bowl.

If you need to water it down further, use a splash of coconut water.

GUT MAKEOVER BREAKFAST CEREAL   ②

(Phase 2)

A handful of blueberries

2 tbsp milled flaxseeds, almonds, Brazil nuts

250ml organic kefir

1 tsp raw honey (optional)
Coconut water (optional)

Mix all the ingredients together in a bowl.

If you wish to water it down further, use a splash of
coconut water.

SPINACH and POTATO   ① ②
SCRAMBLED EGG

Serves 1

The cold potatoes add a prebiotic to this meal, as they are
a resistant-starch food. Although you can still get resistant
starch from reheated cold new potatoes, this does not give
you licence to turn *The Gut Makeover* into a fried chip diet!

1 tbsp extra virgin olive oil
2 small new potatoes, pre-boiled and chilled
A really large handful of spinach, washed
1 large egg, beaten
Sea salt

Heat the oil in a pan over a medium heat. Add the
potatoes and sauté on both sides until golden in colour.

Add the spinach to the pan and cook until it has wilted.

Stir the beaten egg into the potatoes and spinach and
cook, stirring, until the egg is set.

Sprinkle with a little sea salt to your taste and serve.

SCRAMBLED EGGS with SALMON ①②

Serves 1

2 slices of wild Alaskan smoked salmon
1 tbsp extra virgin olive oil (Phase 1) or a knob of butter or
    ghee (Phase 2)
2 eggs, beaten

Cut the slices of salmon into small strips.

Heat the oil or butter or ghee in a pan over a medium heat, add the eggs and salmon and keep stirring until the egg is set and the salmon has changed colour slightly.

WILD SALMON and AVOCADO   ①②

Serves 1

1 ripe avocado, peeled, stoned and sliced
2 slices of wild Alaskan smoked salmon
½ lemon
Freshly ground black pepper, to taste

Arrange the avocado and salmon slices on a plate, squeeze over the juice from the lemon half and season with pepper to taste.

POACHED EGGS and ASPARAGUS ①②

Serves 1

Asparagus contains prebiotic fibres to feed your gut bacteria, and poached eggs are just the nicest way to eat an egg. Usually you see this dish on posh hotel menus, and I've always considered poaching eggs the job of a highly skilled chef. That was until I found out that it is in fact really simple and there are two secret tricks to making a good poached egg. One is vinegar; the other is the use of a small bowl...

Note: Runny eggs can carry salmonella. To avoid this risk do not serve undercooked eggs to the elderly, pregnant women, the very young, or those who are unwell.

2 very fresh eggs
1 tbsp white vinegar, or a light-coloured one such as apple cider vinegar
5 green asparagus spears, wooden ends broken off
Olive oil, for drizzling (Phase 1) or a knob of butter (Phase 2)
Sea salt and freshly ground black pepper, to taste

Boil about 5cm of water in a saucepan and add a tablespoon of vinegar.

Crack one egg into a small bowl and lower the bowl and egg into the pan, then slide the egg gently into the water. Repeat with the other egg.

Put the lid on the saucepan, reduce the heat and simmer for 4 minutes.

Take the eggs out, one at a time, with a slotted spoon and put onto a piece of kitchen paper to drain any excess water.

Meanwhile, steam the asparagus spears for about 5 minutes until they are cooked through and al dente, but not too soft. Remove from the steamer, place on a plate and drizzle with a little olive oil or, if on the second half of the plan, a knob of butter.

Place the poached eggs on top of the asparagus spears, season to taste and serve immediately. The whites of the eggs should be cooked through and the yolks running over the asparagus when you cut into them.

MIDDLE EASTERN RED EGGS   ①②

Serves 2–4

This can make a nice weekend breakfast, or an anytime lunch or dinner. If you make the main sauce, which needs stewing in advance, you can store this in the fridge and just heat it up when you get home from work and throw the eggs in to make a 5-minute meal. Make sure the peppers are well cooked through to make them easier to digest.

3 bell peppers (assortment of colours, e.g. one each of
    red, yellow and green), deseeded and sliced

1 red onion, sliced

3 tbsp virgin olive oil

1 tsp ground cumin

1 tsp harissa paste (available in supermarkets, usually in
  the world food section)

400g tin whole plum tomatoes

3–4 tbsp bone stock of your choice, or water

4 eggs

Sauté the peppers and onion in the olive oil in a frying pan on a medium heat for about 5 minutes until they are softening.

Add the cumin and harissa and stir in, then add the plum tomatoes and break them up with a spoon. Pour in the bone stock or water if the mixture appears too thick. You often need a bit of extra liquid so there is enough moisture for the peppers to stew in, but neither do you want the mixture too watery.

Leave to stew on a low heat for about 30 minutes, or until the peppers are well cooked through and soft.

You can either cool the mixture and store it in the fridge now until a later date when needed, or continue to the next stage.

Make 4 dents into the mixture in the pan and crack in the eggs. Put a lid on and let the eggs steam in the mixture for about 4 minutes if you want them slightly runny in the middle, or 6–7 minutes if you prefer your egg yolks hard.

Serve immediately.

BANANA NUT BREAKFAST BREAD ①②

Makes 1 loaf

Make this at the weekend and have it ready for the mornings over the next week, so you have something delicious to hand when you need to conjure up breakfast quickly. A slice of this is a satisfying accompaniment to one of the shakes if you need more protein in the morning to keep you going. This has been adapted from a recipe by the Nutritional Therapist/Chef Christine Bailey.

2 tbsp extra virgin olive oil
2 cups walnuts
1 cup ground almonds
2 tsp gluten-free baking powder
1 ripe banana
3 large eggs
2 tbsp honey

Grease a loaf tin with a little of the extra virgin olive oil. Preheat the oven to 180°C.

Grind the walnuts in a blender. Add the ground walnuts to the ground almonds and baking powder in a mixing bowl.

Put the banana, eggs, remaining olive oil and honey in the blender and pulse until all broken down. Add the wet mixture to the dry mixture and stir in with a wooden spoon until well combined.

Pour the batter into the loaf tin and bake for 30 minutes, or until a skewer comes out of the mixture clean.

Remove from the oven, turn out and allow to cool on a wire rack.

BANANA and ALMOND BREAKFAST MUFFINS ⑦

Makes 6 muffins

You can make these ahead for the week and store in the fridge for when you need them. The prep time literally takes 5 minutes.

2 ripe bananas
2 eggs
100g butter
1 tbsp honey
200g ground almond flour
1 tsp gluten-free baking powder
1 tbsp raw cacao nibs

Preheat the oven to 180°C. Line a 6-hole muffin tray with paper muffin cases.

Put the bananas, eggs, butter and honey in a blender and pulse to combine.

In a separate bowl, mix the almond flour with the baking powder and cacao nibs.

Add the wet ingredients to the dry, and mix with a wooden spoon. Divide the mixture between the paper cases.

Bake in the oven for about 30 minutes, or until a skewer comes out of the mixture clean. When the muffins are golden on top, and cooked through, take them out to cool down.

CHIA CAVIAR   ①②

This makes a great breakfast served with fresh fruit and scattered with nuts and seeds, but it's equally delicious as a dessert.

240ml unsweetened almond milk or organic kefir (phase 2 only)
2 tbsp chia seeds

Mix the ingredients together in a bowl or large glass and place in the fridge for 2 hours. Every 15 minutes, stir the caviar. You should end up with a soft pearl-like consistency which you can serve alongside either a portion of berries or a couple of slices of fresh mango.

Starters

Starters are a quick and easy way to boost your daily plant intake, and if they contain bitter leaves or fruit, or lemon juice or vinegar they can stimulate the production of stomach acid to help you break your meal down better.

FENNEL GRAPEFRUIT MINT SALAD ①②

Serves 4 as a starter, or 2 as your plants alongside a side of protein with a main meal

Fennel has prebiotic fibres in it to feed your good gut bacteria and the grapefruit is there to trigger your stomach acid to help you break down your forthcoming meal well. Having fennel, onion, grapefruit, mint and olives in one bowl means you shoot up your numbers on your diversity score for the week to help your gut bacteria, too.

1 fennel bulb, cut into fine slivers
1 pear shallot or a small red onion, peeled and cut into
    fine slivers
1 grapefruit (preferably a ruby grapefruit for the colour),
    peeled, deseeded, cut in half then into fine thin strips
2 tbsp chopped fresh mint leaves
4 tbsp walnut oil
2 tbsp Kalamata olives, stoned
Freshly ground black pepper, to taste

Combine all the ingredients in a bowl, toss together and serve immediately.

CRUNCHY RED CHICORY and ① ②
ORANGE SALAD

Serves 2

This makes a delicious starter for two, or you could serve it as a main course lunch for one person with some smoked mackerel.

2 heads red chicory, wooden ends chopped off
100g radishes, stalks cut off and finely sliced (or use 10cm of Chinese white radish (daikon) peeled and finely sliced)
1 small orange, peeled, pips removed and finely sliced
2 tbsp virgin olive oil
1 tbsp apple cider vinegar
Sea salt and freshly ground black pepper, to taste

Assemble the chicory, radishes and orange slices in a serving bowl. Mix the oil, vinegar and seasonings together in a glass, pour over the salad and serve immediately.

SPINACH and RASPBERRY PINE ① ②
NUT SALAD

Serves 2

Handful of cherry tomatoes, halved
Large handful of spinach leaves, washed
¼ red onion, finely chopped
Handful of raspberries (if in season fresh, if not defrosted)

1 tbsp balsamic vinegar

2 tbsp virgin olive oil

1 tbsp pine nuts

Pinch of sea salt

Pinch of chilli flakes

½ tin of anchovies in olive oil, drained

1 tbsp green olives, stoned

Place the tomatoes, spinach and onion in a serving bowl.

In a cup mix the vinegar and oil then add the berries and leave to marinate for 5 minutes in the mixture. Then pour the berries and marinating liquid into the serving bowl with the other ingredients.

Toast the pine nuts in a dry frying pan with the salt and chilli on top for a couple of minutes so they brown.

Throw the toasted nuts, anchovies and olives into the serving bowl with the other ingredients and toss well before serving.

MUSHROOM SOUP ①②

Use organic mushrooms if you can. Mushrooms absorb toxins sprayed on them and from the earth around them, so to avoid risk of exposure to pesticides, use organic.

3 tbsp virgin olive oil

300g organic mushrooms of your choice, washed and
  chopped

½ onion, chopped
1 garlic clove, peeled and chopped
250ml fresh chicken stock
A pinch of sea salt

Heat the oil in a large saucepan and add the mushrooms, onion and garlic and sweat for about 5 minutes on a medium heat.

Add the chicken stock and sea salt and simmer for 15 minutes, then transfer the soup to a blender. Pulse to the texture you like, then serve.

LEEK and SWEET POTATO SOUP   ①②

Serves 4

3 tbsp virgin olive oil
2 leeks, sliced
1 white sweet potato, peeled and cubed (or use the
    orange variety)
250ml home-made chicken stock
500ml water
Sea salt and freshly ground black pepper, to taste

Gently heat the oil in a large saucepan on a medium heat then add the leeks and cook, stirring occasionally, for about 5 minutes until they start to wilt.

Stir in the sweet potato then pour in the chicken stock

and water, season to taste, then raise the heat until the soup is boiling.

Turn down the heat and leave to simmer on a low setting for about 20 minutes until the sweet potatoes are soft.

Pulse the mixture in a blender, then pour into bowls to serve.

JERUSALEM ARTICHOKE and ①② CARROT SOUP

Serves 4

1 onion, peeled and chopped
3 tbsp virgin olive oil
2 cups chopped and peeled Jerusalem artichokes
3 large carrots, chopped and peeled
3 large tbsp home-made chicken stock
250ml water
1 tsp sea salt
Freshly ground black pepper, to taste

Heat the olive oil in a large saucepan and sweat the onion. Add the other vegetables and sweat them with the onion on a low heat for about 5 minutes.

Add the stock and water and season to taste. Simmer for about 30 minutes or until the vegetables are soft.

Transfer the soup to a blender and pulse until smooth.

FIVE NAKED, INSTANT STARTERS

A grapefruit, cut up – choose pink or yellow for variety

An avocado with lemon and Tabasco

A few pieces of fresh chopped pineapple

A radicchio, chopped, with a drizzle of olive oil and balsamic

A handful of rocket leaves with a drizzle of olive oil, balsamic and a little sea salt

Lunches and Dinners

This section gives ideas for making more substantial *Gut Makeover* meals. Some can be knocked up at lunchtime, while others make good evening meals, which in turn can provide delicious leftovers for lunch the next day.

CHICORY and APPLE SALAD ①②

Serves 1

Chicory is a slightly bitter vegetable, so it can stimulate production of your stomach acid to help with digestion. The apples have prebiotic properties to help your gut flora flourish.

2 chicory heads, washed and sliced
1 apple, peeled, cored and sliced
A handful of walnuts, chopped

For the dressing:

Juice of ½ lemon
2 tbsp extra virgin olive oil
1 garlic clove, peeled and finely chopped

Combine all the salad ingredients in a bowl.

Mix the dressing ingredients in a glass with a fork and drizzle over the salad. Serve immediately.

CHICORY and PINE NUT and ROQUEFORT (2)

Serves 2

In the first two weeks, make this salad without the Roquefort. In the second half of the plan, you can add it in to help boost gut bacteria.

140g red or green chicory (about 3 small heads), washed and sliced
1 knob butter
50g pine nuts
A sprinkle of dried chilli flakes, to taste (optional)
A sprinkle of sea salt flakes
2 tbsp extra virgin olive oil

Juice of ½ lemon

Matchbox-sized piece of Roquefort (Phase 2)

Put the chicory in a bowl.

Melt the butter in a frying pan over a medium heat. Add the pine nuts and sprinkle with the chilli flakes, if using, and sea salt. Move the nuts around the pan to coat them well with the butter and flavourings. Cook until the pine nuts are golden brown – watching them carefully as they burn easily.

Sprinkle the warm nuts over the chicory and drizzle with the olive oil and lemon juice. Crumble the cheese over, if using. Serve at once.

MARIO'S ORANGE SALAD   ①②

Serves 2

My Italian friend Mario invited us to his gorgeous shack on the River Thames in London recently while I was writing this book. He's a brilliant cook – home-made pizzas in his 350°C oven being his speciality. We said we'd love to come, then dropped the gluten-free bombshell. Unfazed, Mario conjured up a superb meal and this was his Italian starter, containing the perfect ingredients to stimulate stomach acid production and help digestion. A perfect example of cultural cooking and the real Mediterranean diet that is so good for the gut. This salad was followed by a baked sea bass each.

Use Kalamata olives here, as they are not processed and dyed black like some other varieties.

2 large oranges, peeled, halved and sliced into half moons
1 red onion, thinly sliced into half moons
3 tbsp extra virgin olive oil
2 tbsp Kalamata olives, stoned and chopped
1 small tin of anchovies in olive oil, drained and chopped

Assemble all the ingredients in a salad bowl and serve immediately.

TRIPLE GREENS ①②

Serves 2

It is important to get as much variety of vegetables as possible at every meal, so why include just one vegetable when without much more effort you could eat a triple whammy? This dish is great for getting prebiotic leeks into your diet.

2 tbsp extra virgin olive oil
1cm fresh ginger, peeled and grated or chopped
1 garlic clove, peeled and chopped
1 leek, washed and sliced
170g sugar snap peas, thick tips cut off
100g spinach, washed
A splash of tamari sauce

Heat the oil with the ginger and garlic in a pan. Add the leek and stir until softened. Add the sugar snaps and spinach and stir until the spinach is wilted. Add a splash of tamari sauce and serve.

BUTTERNUT SQUASH and SWEET ①② POTATO SOUP SPRINKLED with CHILLI WALNUTS

Serves 4

This recipe is great for boosting your vitamin A levels. It is the orange pigments in these vegetables that contain vitamin A, which is important for building a strong gut lining, as is the chicken stock, which contains collagen. If you haven't got much fresh stock in your fridge, dilute what you have with boiled water; if you don't have any chicken stock at all, you can just use boiled water. The more stock the better, though, not just for the collagen but also because it will make you feel more full than using just water.

For the soup:

3 tbsp extra virgin olive oil
1 red onion, peeled and chopped
1 garlic clove, peeled and chopped
700g chopped butternut squash and sweet potato (you can buy these in bags, ready chopped, in supermarkets if you need to save time)

500ml fresh chicken stock or water, or a combination of
both
Sea salt and freshly ground black pepper

For the nut topping:
Shelled walnut halves (10 per person)
A sprinkle of dried chilli flakes

Heat the olive oil in a pan and sweat the chopped onion
and garlic until soft and slightly transparent.

Add the butternut squash and sweet potato and sweat
until soft.

Add the stock/water and simmer on a low heat for 20
minutes, partially covered with a lid, until the squash and
sweet potato are soft and break up easily when prodded
with a fork.

Meanwhile, dry-fry the walnuts, sprinkled with a
pinch each of dried chilli flakes and sea salt, until the
nuts are warm and fragrant.

Blitz the soup in a blender, then add salt and freshly
ground pepper to taste. Sprinkle the nuts over the soup
before serving.

ROAST PEPPER and TOMATO SOUP ①②

Serves 4

You could serve this as a starter in the evening to get your vegetable count up, or as a main meal for lunch, with seeds scattered on top for some protein. If you are in the second fortnight of the plan, crumble over a matchbox-sized piece of Roquefort.

5 large tomatoes
2 red bell peppers or sweet red peppers (the long pointy ones)
2 tbsp extra virgin olive oil
1 small onion, chopped
1 garlic clove, peeled and chopped
400ml fresh chicken stock or water, heated
Sea salt and freshly ground black pepper, to taste

Heat the oven to 220°C.

Put the tomatoes and whole peppers on a baking tray and drizzle over 1 tablespoon of the virgin olive oil. Roast in the oven for 20–30 minutes, until the skins are blistering. Remove, then transfer the peppers to a cold saucepan with a lid on and leave to cool for about 15 minutes – this helps the skin to loosen and makes them easier to peel. Peel the peppers and remove the seeds and stalks.

When the tomatoes have cooled down a bit, pinch off the skins.

Heat the remaining olive oil in a pan over a medium heat. Add the onion and garlic and sweat them for about 5 minutes. Stir in the peppers and tomatoes. Add the stock (or water if you don't have any real stock) and simmer for 5–10 minutes over a low heat.

Blitz the mixture in a blender, season to taste and serve.

GAZPACHO ①②

Serves 4

Cold Spanish tomato soup tastes much better than it sounds. It's a kind of Virgin Mary that you can serve as a starter in a cup. Basically, it's a liquidized salad – easy to make and it can be stored in the fridge for a couple of days for a quick down-in-one vegetable boost on the run.

400g tin of tomatoes
½ red onion, chopped
½ medium cucumber
1 garlic clove, peeled and chopped
1 red bell pepper, deseeded and chopped
2 tbsp extra virgin olive oil
1 tbsp red wine vinegar
A dash of Tabasco (optional)
Sea salt and freshly ground black pepper, to taste

Put all the ingredients in a blender and pulse to blend, then store in a jug in the fridge until ready to serve. If the soup is too thick, you can add a little water, or blend in some ice cubes, for a more soupy consistency.

GERMAN POTATO SALAD ①②

Serves 4

If you think potato salad is all gloopy mayonnaise dressings, think again. This version from the south of Germany uses vinaigrette instead, and is naturally perfect gut food – it contains not only prebiotic fibres but also fresh chicken stock for the gut lining. It's important you wait until the potatoes have completely cooled before eating them (even though lukewarm may look enticing), because, when cold, potatoes form a type of fibre called resistant starch, which acts as a prebiotic to feed the beneficial bacteria in your gut. Raw onion gives the salad a nice flavour kick but it also acts as another prebiotic. The chicken stock adds collagen and makes the salad fresh and juicy.

Go easy when serving this salad. Spoon it over about a third of your plate, so that you leave room for lots of colour from other vegetables. This dish goes really well with the Pork Schnitzels (see page 113) and a big half-plateful of steamed fresh asparagus (which also contains its own type of prebiotic fibres).

750g new potatoes, washed and boiled with skins on until
tender

½ white onion, peeled and finely chopped

1 tsp French mustard

4 tbsp extra virgin olive oil

1 tbsp white wine vinegar

½ cup chicken stock (bring this to room temperature if it
is jellified from the fridge, so it is in liquid form)

½ tsp sea salt

Slice the potatoes into thin circles and place in a salad
bowl.

In another bowl, mix together the onion, mustard, oil,
vinegar, stock and salt with a fork, then add this to the
potatoes and let it soak in.

QUICK TIPS FOR CROWDING OUT GRAINS WITH VEGETABLES

A diet featuring a lot of grains can become an irritant
to the gut lining for some people. Many of us eat quite
a large volume of grains over the course of a week, but
actually not in great variety (i.e. we limit ourselves to
just two or three main ones, such as wheat, oats, rice).
During this month we are taking a holiday from grains,
to give the gut a chance to repair. This provides a big
opportunity to use the space left free on the plate,

which we would normally fill with grains, with much more nutrient-dense, gut-friendly foods: vegetables that are teeming with plant chemicals, fibre, vitamins and minerals.

1. **CAULIFLOWER** INSTEAD OF RICE

Cut the hard stalks off a cauliflower and wash and chop the florets into tiny pieces – really shred them or blitz in a food processor.

Sauté the shredded cauliflower in a pan with a drizzle of extra virgin olive oil until soft, then serve with a pinch of salt. You can add chopped fresh herbs, if you like, to make it more tasty, and push up your plant count.

2. **COURGETTE** INSTEAD OF SPAGHETTI

See Courgette Bolognese on page 115. You can either spiralize courgettes into the shape of spaghetti or, if you don't have a spiralizer, simply slice them into half moons, sauté them in extra virgin olive oil and top them with Bolognese sauce.

3. **MIXED ROAST VEGETABLES** INSTEAD OF COUSCOUS

You can buy mixed ready-chopped vegetables in supermarkets, or you could chop up an array of your favourites and bake them in several trays, drizzled with olive oil, in a medium oven until soft. They are delicious eaten immediately, or at room temperature the next day or in packed lunches.

Roast your favourite chopped veg to get a good combination of colours and flavours; my ideal combination is mushrooms, carrots, cauliflower, parsnips, sweet potato, onion and garlic. Squeeze a lemon over the top before serving with a sprinkle of sea salt for extra flavour.

1. USE SWEET POTATOES INSTEAD OF GRAINS

Sweet potatoes contain vitamin A in their orange pigment, which supports your gut lining, so they provide a good nutrient boost instead of grains.

5. USE COLD POTATOES IN MODERATION

Remember, cold potatoes contain resistant starch, which isn't digested in the upper digestive system so it keeps you feeling fuller for longer than hot potatoes. They are useful on one-third of your plate, where you might usually put your grains, but make sure you get lots of colour on the rest of your plate so that there is still a variety of vegetables. We don't want white potatoes becoming the predominant colour, as your gut needs more variety than this.

NIÇOISE SALAD   ①②

Serves 2

For the salad:

1 bag of washed green leaves of your choice

6 herry tomatoes, halved

3 boiled eggs, peeled and quartered

1 tin of tuna in olive oil, drained

1 small bag of flat-leaf parsley, washed and finely chopped

½ red onion, peeled and thinly sliced

100g thin green beans, trimmed, steamed and cooled

2 small cold potatoes

For the dressing:

3 tbsp extra virgin olive oil

1 tbsp freshly squeezed lemon juice or apple cider vinegar

1 garlic clove, roughly chopped

A pinch of sea salt

Toss all the salad ingredients together in a large bowl.

Combine all the dressing ingredients in a cup and stir together well. Pour the dressing over the salad ingredients and serve immediately.

BEETROOT 'HUMMUS' ① ②

Serves 4 as a dip

This tastes delicious smeared on circles of cucumber. If you're on the second half of the plan, it's great spread on a slice of nut 'bread' with a crumble of Roquefort on top.

4 large beetroots, washed
1 garlic clove, peeled and chopped
Juice of 1 lemon
1 tbsp tahini
Sea salt and freshly ground black pepper, to taste

Heat the oven to 180°C.

Roast the beetroots in the oven for about 1 hour, or until tender. Remove from the oven and leave until cool enough to handle, then peel off the skins.

Put the beetroots with all the other ingredients in a blender and blitz until fully combined and a smooth texture. If you prefer a chunkier texture, you can grate the beetroots and mix them with the other ingredients.

CHICORY STUFFED with TUNA   ①②

Serves 2

This can make a quick self-assembly lunch at home, a great starter or an on-the-go packed lunch (just pack the chicory leaves and the filling in separate plastic pots and assemble the dish when you are ready to eat).

16 chicory leaves, washed
1 tin of tuna or sardines in olive oil
1 tbsp capers
1 large gherkin, chopped
Juice of ½ lime
2 globe artichokes, from a tin or jar

Arrange the chicory leaves on a plate.

Mash all the other ingredients together with a fork, including the olive oil from the tins. Divide the mixture between the chicory leaves and serve.

STIR-FRIED SICHUAN GREEN BEANS   ②
with TEMPEH

Serves 1

Sichuan peppers have many different spellings and names (you might see them called Szechuan peppers, or Sichuan flower peppercorns). They taste lemony/peppery and give your whole mouth a really nice buzz (a bit like pins and needles – but nicer!). They are brilliant for cheering up vegetables or tempeh (the fermented soya you can buy in the fridge section or in jars from health-food stores). Sichuan peppers are widely available online and in some supermarkets, such as Sainsbury's. I was first introduced to these peppers by my Chinese sister-in-law, Shuang, who comes from Cheng Du in western China, where they are a staple of the local, widely acclaimed cooking.

200g green beans, topped and tailed
3 tbsp extra virgin olive oil
1 tsp dried chilli flakes
1 tsp Sichuan peppers, crushed or finely chopped
1 tsp ground ginger
1 garlic clove, peeled and finely chopped
½ small white onion, thinly sliced
4 pieces of tempeh, sliced into small pieces
1 tbsp tamari sauce

Wash the green beans, then lay them on a piece of kitchen paper and make sure they are completely dry.

Heat the oil in a wok or frying pan and cook the beans over a medium heat for about 10 minutes until they are a little crinkled and slightly charred. Remove them from the pan and set aside on a plate.

Add the chilli flakes, Sichuan peppers, ginger, garlic and onion to the pan and fry until the onions are melted and moist. Then add the tempeh and stir to coat with the mixture. Toss in the tamari and green beans and serve.

PADRON PEPPERS ①②

Serves 4

Padron peppers are readily available in supermarkets nowadays and they make a wonderful side dish or starter. Eating this dish is a little like playing Russian roulette with your food – you never know when a hot one will strike!

3 tbsp extra virgin olive oil
130g Padron peppers
¼ tsp sea salt

Heat the oil in a pan over a medium heat, add the Padron peppers whole and stir-fry for 5–10 minutes until they are beginning to blister. Serve with sea salt.

CARROT and KEFIR SALAD ②

Serves 4

I've adapted this recipe from a dish I ate at the Huzur Vadisi yoga retreat in Turkey, where I stayed a few years back in a yurt and ate like royalty for a week. The cooked carrots make this salad delicious and nutritious – cooked carrots deliver higher levels of vitamin A than raw ones, which is good news for your gut lining. This is a really convenient salad for packed lunches.

5 large carrots, grated
3 tbsp extra virgin olive oil
½ tsp sea salt
3 tbsp organic kefir
A handful of chopped walnuts
2 garlic cloves, peeled and finely chopped

Sauté the grated carrots in the olive oil in a pan over a medium heat until they turn from a bright orange to a more yellowy orange colour. Stir in the salt.

Wait for the mixture to cool then stir in the kefir, walnuts and garlic and serve at room temperature.

ROASTED BELL PEPPERS ①②

Serves 2

Bell peppers are a wonderful source of vitamin C, which is needed to make energy in the body and supports good skin. Plus, if you use a variety of different colours here, you widen the diversity in your diet to help expand your gut flora. However, some individuals find peppers difficult to digest when they are raw or have the skin on. This recipe gets over these issues and the roasting brings out their sweet flavour.

3 bell peppers – red, yellow and green
Drizzle of extra virgin olive oil
Juice of ½ lemon
A pinch of sea salt

Heat the oven to 230°C.

Put the whole peppers on a baking sheet and bake for 20–30 minutes until the skins are blistering and slightly charred. Remove from the oven and transfer them to a pan and pop the lid on for 15–30 minutes (this makes the skins easier to pull off).

Peel the peppers, cut out the core and seeds and slice the flesh into medium-size strips.

Place the peppers in a bowl and drizzle with a little virgin olive oil, the lemon juice and a pinch of sea salt.

ROASTED TOMATOES with BASIL ①②

When I get home and I need to get my plant count up with minimal work, this is the dish I whip up!

6 tomatoes on the vine
A drizzle of extra virgin olive oil

A sprinkle of sea salt and a grinding of black pepper
Bunch of fresh basil

Heat the oven to 230°C.

Put the tomatoes in a baking dish, drizzle with olive oil, salt and pepper and cook in the oven for about 30 minutes, or until the skins are blistering and the tomatoes look juicy. About 10 minutes before the end, chuck the basil leaves on top and leave them in the oven until they go a little crispy. Whip everything out of the oven and serve.

KEFIR SALAD DRESSING   (2)

We're using fermented milk kefir as well as Roquefort cheese here, for a delicious bacteria laden salad dressing.

80ml organic kefir
Juice of 1 lemon
1 tbsp extra virgin olive oil
A matchbox-sized crumble of Roquefort
A grind of black pepper

Combine all the ingredients in a bowl and mix gently (the cheese can remain a bit crumbled for texture). Pour over any combination of salad.

PERUVIAN CEVICHE   ①②

Serves 4

When I was 19 I went to Lima, Peru, for six months to learn Spanish. At first I was repulsed by the idea of eating raw fish, then I found I craved it when I got back home. In Peru there were *cevicherias* – informal eateries serving nothing but ceviche – all over the place, with ceviche piled high with red onions, limes and chillies, which 'cook' the raw fish. If you like sushi or sashimi and wasabi, you will probably love ceviche.

When I got back from Peru, in 1989, I couldn't find an English cookbook that included this dish or knew of restaurants serving it. Now ceviche is mega popular in big cities and there are English language cookbooks with dozens of versions. This is mine; it's *Gut Makeover* friendly and makes a brilliant dinner-party dish. A nice accompaniment to this dish is some corn on the cobs drizzled in a little butter (if on Phase 2) and salt.

4 pieces of the freshest white fish you can find (about
  200g each), boned and skinned (I usually use cod)
Juice of 6 limes
Juice of 2 lemons
2 Scotch bonnet peppers, deseeded (or regular fresh
  chillies of your choice)
1 medium red onion, finely sliced into half moons

A small bunch of coriander, roughly chopped

1 tbsp sea salt (yes, 1 tablespoon – it gives it a frozen margarita kind of twist)

To serve:

6 sweet potatoes, roasted in their skins for about 1 hour or until soft and juicy, then peeled and chopped in half

Essential kit: a really sharp knife

Lay the pieces of fish on plastic trays or plates and place in the freezer for 1 hour. Whip them out when they are firm, but not frozen through – this makes it easier to cut precise thin slivers. (It's worth planning ahead to include this step – if you don't do this and/or your knife isn't sharp, you can end up with fluffy, rough bits of fish rather than sashimi-style slivers.)

Slice the fish into thin wafers, put them in a bowl and stir in all the remaining ingredients. Within 15 minutes the fish should take on a white 'cooked' appearance.

Serve as soon as possible (marinating the fish for too long can make it mushy). To serve, place the bowl of ceviche in the middle of a platter surrounded with the room-temperature sweet potatoes – the sweet potatoes are the perfect antidote to the sharp, spicy, citrus flavours of the fish.

BAKED SALMON with MUSTARD ①②
and ALMOND CRUST

Serves 2

This is ultra quick and easy to make, and it is also quite an economical dish if you use frozen fish. This is delicious served with a big pile of mixed greens.

2 organic or wild salmon fillets (defrosted if frozen)
2 tbsp French mustard
2 tbsp flaked almonds
A pinch of sea salt
A drizzle of extra virgin olive oil

Heat the oven to 200°C.

Put the salmon on a baking tray then smear mustard on top of each fillet, scatter over the flaked almonds and salt and drizzle over a little olive oil. (This is particularly important if you are using wild Alaskan salmon, as this can be drier than other types.) The almonds should stick onto the fillet to form a nice crust when cooked. Bake in the oven for 20 minutes, or until cooked through.

STEAK NIGHT   ①②

Serves 1

You can vary the steak you use here – organic beef or buffalo, or, if you can get hold of it, use a wild meat such as venison (now sold in supermarkets in fillets, either fresh or frozen), but make sure it is wild and not farmed meat, if possible. To get some colour on your plate, serve this with a pile of mixed roasted vegetables or a large heap of chicory salad.

If you have a large steak or prefer to cook more than one at the same time, you can keep any leftovers in the fridge for the Thai beef salad (see overleaf) the next day.

1 tbsp extra virgin olive oil, ghee or butter
½ onion, thinly sliced
1 fillet of organic steak (beef, buffalo or wild venison)
Sea salt and freshly ground black pepper, to taste

Melt the oil or fat in a frying pan. Add the onion and fry gently until soft and cooked through. Add the steak and sauté gently on both sides until cooked to your liking – you can serve it either raw in the middle or cooked through, depending on your preference. Season with salt and pepper and serve drizzled with the onion and juices from the pan.

THAI BEEF SALAD   ①②

Serves 2

The beauty of a salad like this is that it gets a good variety of vegetables into you in one go, including anti-inflammatory herbs, and also whacks in raw garlic and onion, which are prebiotic and powerful gut-flora boosters. The lemons help with production of stomach acid to aid digestion and absorption of nutrients. Make sure you eat this dish slowly and chew the meat really well.

1 tbsp extra virgin olive oil
240g organic beef steak (such as sirloin) sprinkled with a
    pinch of salt
24 cherry tomatoes, halved
½ cucumber, chopped
½ red onion, peeled and sliced
1 green chilli pepper, chopped, or a red one if you like it
    hotter
2 garlic cloves, peeled and chopped
A large handful of fresh coriander (about 30g), leaves and
    stalks washed and finely chopped
1 tbsp fish sauce
1 tsp tamari sauce
Juice of 2 limes
A few fresh mint leaves, torn (optional)

Heat the olive oil in a frying pan over a medium heat and sauté the steak on both sides. Try not to overcook it – leave it slightly rare in the middle if you like your meat juicy.

When it is cooked to your liking, put the steak on a chopping board and, with a sharp knife, cut off the fat and slice the steak into strips.

While the steak is cooling, put the tomatoes, cucumber, onion, chilli, garlic and herbs into a salad bowl. Add the steak and pour over the fish sauce, tamari and lime juice

Tip the pan juices over the salad and sprinkle on the mint leaves to serve. Mmm.

LEMON and ROSEMARY ①② ROASTED CHICKEN

Serves 4

If you have dismissed the idea of buying a whole organic chicken in the past because you think it is too expensive, think again. You get a lot more for your money if you buy a whole bird rather than breast fillets. If you check the price, a whole organic chicken could be £6.99 a kilo, while a pack of organic breasts is a whopping £20.70 a kilo. You can get maximum value out of one bird by cooking this and the next four recipes.

1 organic chicken
A bunch of fresh rosemary
Juice of ½ lemon

3 tbsp extra virgin olive oil
Sea salt and freshly ground black pepper, to taste

Heat the oven to 160°C.

Remove any elastic bands or string from the chicken. (You want to be able to get the olive oil and herbs into all the crevices to maximise flavour.) Strip the rosemary leaves off the stalks with your hands, then chop them quite finely.

Put the chicken in a roasting tin, then lightly squeeze the lemon juice over and put the squeezed lemon half inside the chicken's cavity. This is key to a juicy, delicious chicken, rather than one that is rubbery and dried out.

Add the rosemary to the olive oil in a small bowl with the salt and pepper. Now pour this over the chicken and massage it into the whole body, especially the legs and wings. This stops the chicken becoming dry when cooking.

Put the chicken in the oven to roast. After 90 minutes, test the chicken to see if it is done – pierce the thigh with the tip of a sharp knife and if the juices run clear, the chicken is cooked. When the chicken is ready, remove it from the oven and leave it to rest for 15 minutes, covered with a piece of tin foil.

When serving the chicken, make sure each portion comes drizzled with a generous scoop of the delicious lemon/rosemary-flavoured gelatinous juices, which should have formed at the bottom of the pan.

WARM GREEN CHICKEN SALAD   ①②

Serves 1

Pouring a warm red onion and red wine vinegar dressing over this salad gives it a delightfully sweet and sour flavour.

2 huge handfuls of baby spinach leaves, washed
1 huge handful of rocket leaves, washed
½ tin of anchovies in olive oil, drained and chopped
The leftover chicken picked off the leg of a roast chicken
3 tbsp extra virgin olive oil
1 red onion, peeled and chopped
2 large garlic cloves, peeled and chopped
2 tbsp red wine vinegar

Combine the salad leaves, anchovies and chicken in a salad bowl.

Heat the olive oil in a pan over a medium heat, add the onion and garlic and sauté until they are soft and slightly transparent. Take off the heat, wait a minute, then add the red wine vinegar. Pour this mixture over the salad and serve at once.

MULTI-COLOURED MISO ② CHICKEN STIR-FRY

Serves 2

Unpasteurised fermented miso – the paste, not the freeze-dried stuff – is a good alternative probiotic food if you can't tolerate kefir. It can be found in the fridge of good health-food stores and Asian supermarkets.

3 tbsp extra virgin olive oil

1 garlic clove, peeled and chopped

2cm fresh ginger, peeled and chopped

450g bag of vegetable stir-fry mix (e.g. beansprouts, broccoli, onions, cabbage, carrots)

1 courgette, sliced (to add bulk, remember no rice!)

A handful of chopped chicken from your leftover roast chicken

1 cup fresh chicken stock (see page 184)

1 tbsp fish sauce

A sprinkle of tamari sauce

1 tbsp fermented miso

Heat the oil in a frying pan and stir-fry the garlic and ginger on a medium heat for about 2 minutes. Add all the vegetables and stir-fry for about 5 minutes. Add the chicken and chicken stock and stir in.

Cook, stirring occasionally, until the broccoli is al dente (not rock hard, but not limp).

Sprinkle on the fish sauce and tamari to taste, then stir in the miso and serve immediately.

ASIAN-STYLE GUT-HEALING SOUP ②

Serves 1

This is perfect for Phase 1 of the plan because chicken stock provides collagen which can help heal the gut lining, and the salmon contains omega-3 essential fatty acids to help reduce gut inflammation (if this is an issue). The pak choi (prebiotic) and fermented miso (probiotic) work in concert to boost gut flora. The first time you try the miso, you may like to start with a quarter teaspoon, or a half, and build up the amount as your gut gets used to it.

A knob of coconut oil
1 garlic clove, peeled and chopped
1cm fresh ginger, peeled and chopped
2 spring onions, sliced
120g organic or wild salmon, cubed
2 pak choi, washed and sliced
250ml fresh chicken stock (see page 184)
1 tsp fresh fermented miso
Juice of 1 lime
1 tsp tamari sauce
1 tsp fish sauce

Heat the coconut oil in a frying pan or wok on medium heat and sauté the garlic, ginger and spring onions. Add the salmon and cook through. Add the pak choi and stir around until just beginning to wilt. Add the chicken stock and heat through. Then add the rest of the ingredients, including the miso, and take off the heat (so the bacteria in the miso are not killed off by high temperature cooking) and then serve.

LEBANESE LEMON CHICKEN LIVERS ①②
and POMEGRANATE

Serves 2

I'm always looking for quick, easy and palatable ways to cook organ meats and I came across this combination in a Lebanese restaurant while on holiday in Egypt. Liver contains a form of vitamin A which is needed to build a strong gut lining, and this form is more absorbable than that found in the orange pigment of vegetables such as butternut squash and pumpkins. This form is also found in egg yolks and real butter. Some supermarkets now sell organic livers and also pomegranate molasses in bottles.

4 tbsp extra virgin olive oil
1 red onion, thinly sliced in half moons
1 garlic clove, peeled and sliced
400g organic chicken livers

A knob of butter (Phase 2)

2 tbsp pomegranate molasses

Juice of 1 lemon

50g fresh watercress

Sea salt and freshly ground black pepper, to taste

Heat the oil in a pan on a medium heat and gently sauté the onion and garlic until soft. Add the livers and sauté gently – if you want them tender and slightly pink in the middle, whip them off the heat soon after they change colour; if you like them cooked through, leave them slightly longer, but just a couple more minutes otherwise they can become tough. If you're on the second part of the programme, stir in the butter when the livers are cooked.

Stir in the pomegranate molasses then add the lemon juice, salt and pepper.

Pile the watercress leaves onto a plate, top with the livers, then pour the juices over and enjoy.

PORK SCHNITZELS   ①②

Serves 4

This is great with two other gut-boosting accompaniments – the German Potato Salad on page 90, and a pile of steamed asparagus. If you are buying your meat from a butcher, ask him or her to stamp each fillet with a meat tenderizer hammer so they are nice and thin and the meat is more tender and easy to digest. If you are buying the meat in a supermarket ready packaged, you could use the steaks as they come (about 1cm thick), or buy a meat tenderizer (about £5) and hammer them yourself to make them less chewy.

English mustard bought as a paste normally contains gluten but the powder doesn't, so it's OK to use it in this recipe. Arrowroot is usually found in the baking section of supermarkets.

200g ground almonds
1 tsp English mustard powder
2 tbsp arrowroot
1 tsp paprika
½ tsp cayenne pepper
1 tsp sea salt
120ml extra virgin olive oil
4 organic pork loin steaks (total weight 500g)

Heat the oven to 220°C.

Combine the ground almonds, mustard powder, arrowroot, paprika, cayenne pepper and sea salt in a shallow bowl.

Pour the olive oil into a separate shallow bowl.

Dip each piece of pork into the oil then dip it into the almond mixture to coat it on both sides. Place on a baking tray and cook the schnitzels in the oven for 20 minutes until golden brown.

COURGETTE BOLOGNESE   ①②

Serves 8

I've been cooking this for years, first in a big pot, which would hiss and steam on the hob for hours, but more recently in a pressure cooker in just 30 minutes. Don't limit yourself to beef for tradition's sake; it's important to use a variety of proteins in the diet to expose ourselves to a range of different nutrients, so go beyond beef in your Bolognese. Minced meat should be easy to digest and absorb because not only has it been minced, as the name suggests, but it has been well cooked, too.

If you make this sauce in bulk like this, you can freeze leftovers in small portions for another day.

4 tbsp extra virgin olive oil

1 large onion (or 2 small ones), finely chopped

4 garlic cloves, peeled and chopped

2 celery sticks, finely chopped

1kg organic beef, buffalo or lamb mince

2 x 400g tins whole plum tomatoes

140g tomato purée

4 tbsp fresh chicken stock (see page 184)

A bunch of fresh rosemary, washed and leaves finely
    chopped

1 tsp sea salt

For the courgette 'spaghetti':

1 medium courgette per person

1 tbsp extra virgin olive oil

A pinch of sea salt

Heat the oil in a pan (or pressure cooker pot, if you prefer) on a medium heat and sauté the onion, garlic and celery. Add the mince and cook until browned, stirring occasionally.

Add the tomatoes and tomato purée, chicken stock, rosemary and salt and stir, gently breaking up the plum tomatoes with a wooden spoon.

Cook on a low heat with the lid slightly ajar for 3–4 hours, or cook according to the manufacturer's instructions for 30 minutes in a pressure cooker.

When ready to eat, top and tail the courgettes and turn them through a spiralizer. If you don't have a spiralizer, slice the courgettes into half moons. Put a tablespoon of olive oil in a pan, add the courgettes and cook for a few minutes until softened – half-moon shapes may need a little longer. Season with a pinch of sea salt.

Serve the cooked courgette on individual plates, topped with a portion of Bolognese sauce.

MEDITERRANEAN ROAST VEGETABLES ①②

Serves 2

This is a good way of filling a large portion of your plate with a variety of different vegetables. The combination here is just a suggestion – you probably have your own favourites. If you're short of time, you can cheat by buying bags of ready chopped vegetables from supermarkets and roasting them drizzled with a little extra virgin olive oil and sea salt.

1 large red onion, cut into eighths
1 large courgette, trimmed, cut into three widthways, then
    eighths lengthways
1 yellow pepper, deseeded and cut into eighths
20 cherry tomatoes
4 tbsp extra virgin olive oil
Sea salt and freshly ground black pepper, to taste

Heat the oven to 160°C.

Tip all the ingredients into a roasting tin and mix together well. Slow-roast in the oven for 50 minutes until softened and juicy.

MEATBALLS IN PAPRIKA and CAYENNE TOMATO SAUCE   ①②

Serves 4

Meatballs make a hearty meal and are often good heated or eaten at room temperature the next day. If you set some meatballs aside after cooking and don't add sauce, you can keep these as a convenient protein addition to an easy-to-eat packed lunch.

500g minced meat (lamb, beef, pork or a mixture of two of these)
A handful of fresh flat-leaf parsley, chopped
1 egg
4 garlic cloves, peeled and finely chopped
1 tsp smoked sweet paprika

For the sauce:

2 tbsp extra virgin olive oil
4 red onions, finely chopped
1 garlic clove, peeled and finely chopped
2 tsp cayenne pepper
1 tsp smoked sweet paprika
2 x 400g tins of whole plum tomatoes
Sea salt and freshly ground black pepper, to taste

Heat the oven to 200°C.

Mix the meat, parsley, egg, garlic and sweet paprika in a bowl. Put spoonfuls into the palm of your hand and roll them into balls or small patties.

Place them on a baking tray in rows, slightly spaced apart, and bake for about 20 minutes, until cooked through.

Meanwhile, make the sauce. Heat the olive oil in a pan on a medium heat and sauté the onions and garlic for 5 minutes, then add the cayenne pepper, paprika and plum tomatoes, breaking up the tomatoes with a spoon. Season to taste and leave to simmer for 15 minutes.

When the meatballs are done, add them to the sauce and cook for 5 minutes. Serve with a large green salad with avocados and nuts.

SPANISH MEATBALLS IN ALMOND SAUCE ①②

Serves 4

We normally think about meatballs going well with tomato sauces, but almond sauces, which are popular in Spanish cooking, are delicious and nutritious, too.

500g minced pork
1 small onion, finely chopped
1 garlic clove, peeled and finely chopped
½ tsp sea salt

Freshly ground black pepper, to taste

A grating of nutmeg

1 egg

1 tbsp ground almonds

3 tbsp extra virgin olive oil

For the almond sauce:

3 tbsp extra virgin olive oil

2 garlic cloves, peeled and finely chopped

4 tbsp ground almonds

1 tsp hot smoked paprika

½ tsp each salt and ground black pepper

200ml thick, gelatinous chicken stock (add a little water if
    you need to make the sauce a little thinner)

Put all the meatball ingredients, except the olive oil, in a
bowl and mix them together. Put spoonfuls into the palm
of your hand and roll them into small balls.

Heat the olive oil in a pan on a medium heat, add the
meatballs and pan-fry until they are lightly browned.
Keep turning them every couple of minutes so they cook
through properly. Set aside and make the almond sauce.

In a clean pan, heat the olive oil on a medium heat.
Add the garlic and fry until golden, then add the ground
almonds, hot smoked paprika, salt and pepper. Stir in the
chicken stock then add the meatballs. Leave to cook over
a low heat for about 5 minutes while the sauce thickens.

SEA BASS with SALSA VERDE ①②

Serves 4

This is an ultra-quick meal for after work and provides good leftovers, too! The salsa verde can be used the next day to accompany other dishes or as a dressing for a salad, thinned down with more virgin olive oil. Serve with a large portion of green salad or steamed spinach on the side.

4 sea bass fillets, with skin on
1 tbsp extra virgin olive oil
Sea salt and freshly ground black pepper, to taste

The sauce:
A handful of fresh basil
A handful of fresh parsley
1 tbsp capers
4 tinned anchovy fillets, drained
4 tbsp extra virgin olive oil
1 tbsp Dijon mustard
1 garlic clove, peeled and chopped

Place all the sauce ingredients in a blender and blitz in short bursts until the main ingredients are broken down but the mixture is still rough and textured. Set aside.

Lightly season the fish. Heat the oil in a frying pan over a medium heat then place the fish skin-side down in the pan and cook over a medium heat until the skin is crispy. Turn over and cook for a couple of minutes on the other side until cooked through.

Serve the fish with a drizzle of the salsa verde on top.

BUN-LESS BURGER and SWEET POTATO WEDGES ①②

Serves 4

When it comes to burgers, I'm a great believer in simplicity and quality. That's why the meat speaks for itself here and the condiments sing the chorus. The wedges can be dunked in the raw tomato ketchup on page 129.

For the burger:

500g beef or buffalo mince

½ small white onion, finely chopped

A small handful of fresh flat-leaf parsley, finely chopped

1 egg

Extra virgin olive oil, for frying

A small slice of Roquefort cheese per burger (Phase 2)

1 tomato, sliced

4 slices of gherkin

Sea salt and freshly ground black pepper, to taste

For the wedges:

4 medium-sized sweet potatoes, peeled and cut into
   wedges

4 tbsp extra virgin olive oil
A sprinkle of cayenne pepper
A sprinkle of paprika
½ tsp sea salt

Heat the oven to 200°C.

First get the potatoes in the oven. Lay the wedges on a large baking tray and sprinkle with the oil, cayenne pepper, paprika and salt. Stir the ingredients together with your hands or a spoon so they are all coated in the mixture. Cook in the oven for 40 minutes or until golden. Halfway through the cooking time, take the potatoes out and tussle them around so the other sides are exposed and can crisp up.

While the potatoes are cooking, make the burgers. Using a wooden spoon, mix the meat with the onion, parsley, egg and salt and pepper to taste, then split the mixture into four and form into round burger shapes with your hands.

Put a little olive oil in a frying pan, then cook the burgers on a medium heat for about 5 minutes, until they are lightly browned, then turn them over and keep cooking until they are cooked through. Near the end, put a slice of Roquefort on top and let it melt into the top of the burger (Phase 2 only).

Serve a burger on each plate with a slice of tomato and gherkin on top and the sweet potato wedges on the side. Serve with the raw ketchup on page 129.

GUT MAKEOVER 'BREAD'   ①②

I thought long and hard before including this recipe, as nuts and seeds eaten in bulk can mean a large amount of fat in one sitting. Although *The Gut Makeover* includes beneficial fats as needed in cooking to make it taste good, and to make us feel full, they do need to be kept in check so that a meal isn't dominated by them.

We're aiming for the vegetables and colour to take centre stage in every meal, so enjoy a slice of this toasted, with a smear of miso paste on top, or some roasted artichokes from a jar, or some beetroot hummus, or with roasted peppers and a squeeze of lemon and maybe a little cayenne pepper and a large side salad, to keep your plant count up. This recipe is an adaptation from one by Danish celebrity chef Thomas Rode.

3 cups walnuts, roughly chopped
2 cups almonds, roughly chopped
2 cups mixed seeds, e.g. pumpkin seeds, sunflower seeds, flaxseeds
5 eggs, beaten
80ml extra virgin olive oil, plus extra for greasing
1 tsp sea salt

Heat the oven to 160°C. Grease a loaf tin with olive oil.
Mix the nuts and seeds together in a bowl. In another

bowl, mix together the eggs, oil and sea salt. Stir the wet and dry ingredients together.

Transfer the mixture to the greased loaf tin and bake in the oven for 1 hour. Remove from the oven and leave to cool in the tin before cutting into slices.

When cooled, store, wrapped, in the fridge, to keep it fresh for longer.

WARNING: HEALTHY BEHAVIOURS ARE INFECTIOUS

I recently worked with a company of 40 staff in London on a workplace wellness programme. The CEO was proud that her staff represented 15 different nationalities, the point being that talent was recruited from all over the world, and the company was a culturally rich place to work. I noticed immediately that around 80 per cent of the staff were bringing in delicious leftovers, from multi-coloured, vegetable-count-high curries to Bolognese, and eating them at tables in a communal kitchen. These staff members were not only saving money by doing this but supporting their health, too.

So the starting point for improving this group's eating habits was several notches above anywhere else I have been, where the status quo is often poor-quality sandwiches eaten at desks. Infectious behaviours are important when it comes to developing healthy behaviours; if you work around others who are eating low-nutrient, beige-coloured food at their desks, you are more likely to do so too. If you hang around with people who cook proper evening meals and bring in leftovers the next day and move away from their desks to eat it, you are also likely to – and others may even join you!

I recommend doing *The Gut Makeover* with a buddy if you can find one. You can support one another, but you may also find your new eating habits and behaviours start to spread to other colleagues, too.

HOW TO ASSEMBLE A GUT MAKEOVER PACKED LUNCH

Many of the recipes in this book provide great leftovers for lunch the next day – anything from curry with cauliflower rice to Bolognese with courgette spaghetti. Sometimes slow-cooked foods just taste even better the next day.

If you have a microwave or oven at work you could heat up the leftovers for lunch – if you are using a microwave, empty your lunch onto a ceramic plate first and heat on this to avoid microwaved plastic leaching into your food.

I prefer my packed lunches at room temperature; in most UK weather, you don't need to worry about your food going off between coming out of your fridge in the morning and being eaten five hours later at lunch.

All of the following lunch ideas can be eaten cold or at room temperature. See the section overleaf on dressings, dips and sauces if you want to jazz up these dishes.

It's a good idea to invest in some portable, non-spill containers to transport your lunch in. Choose a box with a lid for the main ingredients below and a separate, smaller, lidded one for sauces, dips or dressings.

Protein	Load up with plants
Smoked mackerel bought ready to eat	Ready cooked beetroots and washed chicory leaves go really well with this. Add French dressing and a small, cold white potato.
Steak	Bag of mixed salad leaves (the more varieties the better, e.g. lamb's lettuce, rocket and watercress). A small, cold white potato. A drizzle of pesto, mixed with extra virgin olive oil, over the lot.

Roast chicken leg	A big pile of roasted vegetables. The raw ketchup goes nicely with these and the meat.
2 boiled eggs, ½ tin of tuna and some anchovies	Chopped tomatoes, cucumbers, red onions, Kalamata olives and a vinaigrette dressing.
Wild Alaskan salmon	Sliced ripe avocado, pieces of celery and radishes with a drizzle of extra virgin olive oil and a teaspoon of balsamic vinegar.
Pork schnitzel	German potato salad and a large pile of steamed green asparagus.

Bring a piece of fruit for dessert, as this automatically bumps up your plant count for the day.

Dressings, dips and sauces

Some people say they don't eat many vegetables each day because they find them boring or not particularly tasty. The way to jazz up vegetables and make sure they taste good is to have delicious dressings, dips and sauces to hand. These often provide the bridge to vegetables and hence a better diet.

Here are three simple additions that can be easily put together to liven up most lunch-box combinations.

1. **Pesto** – Put into a blender: a large handful of fresh basil leaves, about 80ml of extra virgin olive oil, the juice of one lemon, a handful of pine nuts and a little salt. Make it quite runny so it acts as a nice cold sauce you can drizzle over cold meats, fish and salads or roast vegetables.

2. **Raw ketchup** – Put into a blender: half a jar of sun-dried tomatoes (about 150ml – you can buy them in jars, packed in oil) with two tablespoons of extra virgin olive oil, two large fresh tomatoes, half a red onion, a garlic clove, a handful of fresh basil and a little sea salt. Add enough extra virgin olive oil to make the sauce the consistency of tomato ketchup. This is absolutely delicious and great for the gut flora because the onions and garlic are raw rather than cooked.

3. **Simple French dressing** – Stir together three parts extra virgin olive oil to one part red wine vinegar with a teaspoon of French mustard and a little sea salt and pepper. The mustard not only tastes good but also binds together the other ingredients.

FIVE AFTER-WORK SUPERMARKET QUICK
GUT MAKEOVER MEALS

1. **Starter:** Bag of **rocket** (add drizzle of extra virgin olive oil and splash of balsamic vinegar)

Main: Bag of **spiralized butternut squash** (now widely available in supermarkets)

Defrosted **Bolognese sauce** (see page 115 – you can make this from lamb, beef or turkey mince)

2. **Starter:** 2 heads of **chicory** chopped and served with drizzle of extra virgin olive oil and splash of apple cider vinegar. Sprinkle with seeds of your choice and a little sea salt

Main: a bag of **root vegetables to bake** bought in the supermarket, such as ready chopped pumpkin and sweet potato – whatever combination is available. Roast in the oven for about 25 minutes, drizzled in a little olive oil, some sea salt and, if you like, some chilli flakes

Stick a **piece of salmon** under the grill with some seasoning on top and serve with squeezed lemon dressing and some chopped herbs

3. **Starter: a grapefruit** (cut in half and spoon out segments)

Main: A **sirloin steak** gently fried on both sides to your liking in a little extra virgin olive oil and some seasoning, alongside **a large bag of salad** with balsamic and extra virgin olive oil drizzled on top. Add extra tomatoes, radishes, olives, spring onions – whatever you have time to add

4. **Starter:** a cup of **chicken stock** with a little seasoning and a squeeze of lemon

Main: A **vegetable stir-fry** – gently fry a little chopped and peeled ginger, garlic and spring onion in a pan. Add a packet of **prawns or cashew nuts**. Then throw a whole bag of supermarket fresh stir-fry mix and toss until it wilts. Add a splash of tamari sauce and fish sauce. If using egg as your protein, whisk in a bowl and add this near the end of the cooking time

5. **Starter:** a bowl of **ready chopped fresh pineapple**

Main: A supermarket warm **ready-roasted chicken**. Separately pan-fry **a big pile of veg**, e.g. a chopped courgette and a little onion, then add a large handful of frozen peas. Add a couple of spoons of your chicken stock, half a squeezed lemon, some chopped parsley and a little seasoning, and serve

Plants

ROAST PARSNIP and CARROT CHIPS ①②

Serves 4

5 parsnips, peeled and cut into roughly equal-size chips
2 carrots, peeled and cut into roughly equal-size chips
4 tbsp virgin olive oil
A sprinkle of cayenne pepper
Sea salt and freshly ground black pepper, to taste

Heat the oven to 200°C.

Combine all the ingredients in a shallow baking dish and bake for about 30 minutes (cooking time will depend on how thick or thin you have cut your chips). Check on them from time to time and turn so they get evenly cooked. Remove when they are cooked through and the edges are slightly crisp.

SWEDE MASH   ①②

Serves 4

In some countries the root vegetable swede is considered animal feed, not good enough for human consumption. I can't understand this; it is absolutely delicious and very cheap, too. This makes a good alternative to traditional potato mash while on *The Gut Makeover* plan.

1 swede, peeled and cubed

2 tbsp extra virgin olive oil or a large knob of butter
 (Phase 2)

1 garlic clove, peeled and finely chopped

2cm fresh ginger, peeled and grated

Sea salt and freshly ground black pepper, to taste

Either steam or boil the swede in a puddle of water until it is soft (roughly 30 minutes – the smaller the cubes, the quicker the cooking time). Drain, and reserve a little of the cooking water.

Heat the oil or butter in a pan then add the garlic and ginger and sweat on a medium heat for about 5 minutes.

Put the swede, with a little of the reserved cooking water, in a blender with the oil/butter mixture and salt and pepper to taste. Blitz quickly, but not for too long, so that it retains a bit of texture.

SWEET and SOUR KALE and APPLE SALAD ①②

Serves 2

I'm a bit biased against kale. It conjures up too many images of holier-than-thou eating programmes and, quite frankly, I've always found it repulsive when cooked or steamed. That was until a client, Natalie, told me she went to Copenhagen and had the most amazing kale and apple salad with an apple cider dressing.

This is my concoction, and I can't quite believe it myself, but I can eat masses of this and enjoy every mouthful. I find it tastes so much better than cooked kale because the dressing soaks in and gives it a really nice flavour. Real maple syrup is pricey, but it is easy to mix into a dressing because it is easy to pour. You could use raw honey instead, though it's trickier to bind.

½ a bag of fresh kale, washed, hard stems torn off and
     leaves finely shredded
1 apple, cored and cut into small pieces
1 avocado, peeled, stoned and cut into small pieces
1 tbsp fresh pomegranate seeds

For the dressing:
4 tbsp extra virgin olive oil
2 tbsp apple cider vinegar
1 tbsp maple syrup
½ small red onion, finely chopped
1 tsp Dijon mustard
½ tsp sea salt

Assemble all the plants in a salad bowl.

In a jar, combine the dressing ingredients (putting the red onion in this mixture imparts more flavour in the dressing and helps to emulsify the dressing).

Pour the dressing over the salad and toss thoroughly, so the leaves really soak up the dressing, and serve immediately.

SPINACH and PINE NUTS   ①②

Serves 2 as a side dish

4 tbsp extra virgin olive oil
260g bag of spinach leaves, washed
1 tbsp flat-leaf parsley, chopped
4 anchovies, chopped
50g pine nuts
Sea salt and freshly ground black pepper, to taste

Heat the olive oil in a pan on a medium heat.

Add the spinach leaves and stir from time to time until the leaves have wilted.

Scatter the parsley on top, then stir in the anchovies, pine nuts and seasoning.

STICKY JERUSALEM ARTICHOKES   ①②
with GARLIC and BAY LEAVES

Serves 4 as a side dish

Adapted from a recipe by Jamie Oliver, this is a delicious injection of prebiotics into your gut. The cooked artichokes also taste good at room temperature the next day.

600g Jerusalem artichokes, peeled and cut into quarters
4 tbsp extra virgin olive oil

8 bay leaves
2 garlic cloves, peeled and chopped
1 tbsp apple cider vinegar
Sea salt and freshly ground black pepper, to taste

Place the artichokes in a pan with the olive oil on a medium heat and gently sauté them. They should sizzle away, becoming a little golden on each side.

Add the bay leaves and garlic.

Reduce the heat, put on a lid and let them cook for about another 20 minutes until they are cooked through and soft, but sticky and golden on the outside.

Add the vinegar and seasoning and serve straight away.

STIR-FRIED TAT SOI   ①②

Serves 2

I've recently noticed some supermarkets selling tat soi – which provides another great opportunity for some diversity. It's similar to pak choi in flavour, but with longer, thinner stalks and smaller leaves. Sichuan peppers can usually be found in the spice section of a shop and have a lemony flavour which is highly addictive once you've tried it.

1 garlic clove, peeled and chopped
2cm fresh ginger, peeled and chopped

1 tsp of Sichuan peppers, crushed (I just lean a heavy knife
    on top of them on a chopping board)

3 tbsp extra virgin olive oil

2 large stalks of tat soi, chopped into three (you should end up
    with three short sticks from each stem, including the leaf)

A splash of tamari sauce

Sauté the garlic, ginger and Sichuan peppers in the olive oil on a medium heat until the vegetables start to sweat, then add the tat soi and cook until they are wilted.

    Add a splash of tamari and serve.

AROMATIC STEWED ①②
PAPRIKA TOMATOES

Serves 4 as a side dish

This is a good dish to make in advance to have in the fridge for after work as a side dish, or you can freeze it.

1 onion, chopped

1 garlic clove, peeled and chopped

2 tbsp extra virgin olive oil

2 x 400g tins whole plum tomatoes

1 tsp paprika

½ tsp ground cumin

½ tsp sea salt

A handful of chopped fresh flat-leaf parsley, to serve

Sauté the onion and garlic in the olive oil in a saucepan on a medium heat, then add the tomatoes and spices. Lower the heat and simmer for 45 minutes with the lid half on.

Scatter the parsley on top before serving.

ROASTED SWEET POTATOES   ①②

Serves 2

2 large orange-coloured sweet potatoes
5 tbsp extra virgin olive oil
1 tsp sea salt and a grinding of black pepper, to taste

Put the sweet potatoes into a wide oven dish. Drizzle over the olive oil and toss the sweet potatoes so they are well covered.

Add the seasoning.

Bake in the oven on 220°C, stirring from time to time, for about 25 minutes, till cooked through and a little crisp on top.

RATATOUILLE   ①②

Serves 4

This stew freezes well and can be cooked ahead, stored in the fridge and then spooned out and heated up at short notice as a side to a piece of meat or fish.

3 tbsp extra virgin olive oil

1 red onion, chopped

3 garlic cloves, peeled and finely chopped

1 yellow bell pepper, deseeded and cut into cubes

1 aubergine, cut into cubes

2 courgettes, cut into cubes

400g tin whole plum tomatoes

1 tbsp tomato purée

100ml water or fresh chicken stock

Sea salt and freshly ground black pepper, to taste

Heat the olive oil in a pan over a medium heat. Add the onion, garlic and bell pepper. After about 5 minutes, when the onions are beginning to look transparent, add the aubergine and courgettes and let them sizzle gently for about 5 minutes, stirring regularly.

Add the tomatoes, the purée and, if needed, the water or stock and stir in, breaking up the tomatoes with a wooden spoon.

Season to taste and leave to cook over a low heat with a lid on for 60–90 minutes until you have a rich, glossy vegetable stew.

AUBERGINE CAVIAR with RED ①② CHICORY LEAVES

Serves 4

This is a recipe I've made and enjoyed many times since learning it from the French chef René Bérard, at Hostellerie Bérard, in Provence. The roasted garlic and aubergine taste delicious together and make a great alternative to chickpea hummus over these four weeks.

4 aubergines
Extra virgin olive oil, for drizzling
A sprinkling of dried thyme
8 garlic cloves, skin on
3 basil leaves, thinly sliced
Sea salt and freshly ground black pepper, to taste
A sprinkle of cayenne pepper

To serve:
4 red chicories, the hard end chopped off, leaves
   separated

Heat the oven to 220°C.
   Remove the stems from the aubergines. Cut the aubergines in half lengthways, score the flesh in a crisscross pattern and place the halves in a baking dish. Drizzle with the olive oil and sprinkle with some salt, pepper and thyme.

Place a garlic clove on top of each piece of aubergine.

Bake in the oven for about 1 hour until they are going golden and the flesh is soft.

Remove the aubergine flesh with a spoon and place it in a blender. Pulse until smooth, then add the basil.

Sprinkle over some cayenne pepper to serve, then place the aubergine caviar in a bowl at room temperature in the middle of a table, with a pile of red chicory leaves to eat the dip with.

COOKED CARROT and ①② CORIANDER SALAD

Serves 4

Vitamin A, one of the nutrients needed for a healthy gut lining, is found in carrots and needs to be eaten with some oil or fat to be absorbed by the body. This is a typical Middle Eastern dish which combines olive oil and cooked carrots; interestingly, it is easier to absorb vitamins from cooked carrots than raw. It tastes gorgeous eaten at room temperature in packed lunches or as a side to grilled meat or fish, and lasts well in the fridge for a couple of days. I also like making it because I don't have to grate raw carrots and risk grazing my hands, which is often the case with carrot salads!

500g carrots, peeled
½ tsp ground cumin
1 garlic clove, peeled and finely chopped
½ tsp sea salt
Juice of 1 lemon
1 tbsp extra virgin olive oil
A handful of fresh coriander, finely chopped

Boil or steam the whole carrots in water with a pinch of salt until they are just tender. Drain, then put under cold running water to cool. Leave to drain, then thinly slice the carrots.

Heat the ground cumin in a pan for a couple of minutes and stir until it emits a lovely aroma, as if it's roasting.

Transfer the cumin to a small bowl and stir in the sea salt and the chopped garlic, then add the lemon juice and olive oil.

Put the carrots in a serving bowl, pour over the dressing and chopped coriander and toss well.

Serve at room temperature.

KEFIR COURGETTES   ②

Serves 4

Super simple to make and delicious, too. This recipe gives good leftovers, and the Middle Eastern sumac and za'atar spices (which are now widely available in UK supermarkets) make this dish sing. You can use cow's milk kefir or, if you have it – or have made it – goat's milk kefir tastes particularly tangy in this dish.

4 courgettes, cut into 2cm slices
2 tbsp extra virgin olive oil
200ml organic kefir
Juice of ½ lemon
1 tsp sumac
Sea salt, to taste
A sprinkling of za'atar

Sauté the courgettes in the olive oil in a frying pan on a medium heat until all the medallions are blistered on both sides.

Remove from the heat and put in a bowl.

Pour over the kefir and lemon juice, then sprinkle on the sumac, salt and za'atar and serve at room temperature.

HARISSA POTATO SALAD   ①②

Serves 4

This goes well with the pickled lemon sea bass, carrots with coriander and/or kefir courgettes (see pages 150, 141 and opposite). Wonderful for packed lunches and leftovers.

750g new potatoes
1 tsp harissa paste
3 tbsp virgin olive oil
Juice of 1 lemon
Sea salt, to taste

Wash and boil the potatoes in their skins in a pan of simmering water until soft but still slightly firm inside when tested with a fork (about 20 minutes, depending on the size of the potatoes).

Drain the potatoes, then set them under cold running water to cool them down so you can handle them. Drain, then cut all the potatoes into slices with their skin on (life's too short to peel new potatoes!).

In a cup mix the harissa, olive oil, lemon juice and sea salt.

Pour the dressing over the potatoes and let it sink in – it should become a lovely reddish golden colour from the harissa and the olive oil. When cooled down, enjoy!

PERUVIAN POTATO SALAD   ②

My influence for creating this is a dish called Papa a la Huancaína, from the Andes in Peru. This is a distant relative, using gut-friendly kefir rather than the evaporated milk you see in the usual recipes. The key to its deliciousness is to use really good-quality speciality potatoes. In the UK, Jersey Royals (when in season) work well, or I've found some supermarkets now selling small trays of mixed-coloured potatoes – with purple, yellow and red. Purple potatoes, with their dark colour, would deliver polyphenols to feed your beneficial gut bacteria, as well as resistant starch fibres formed from the potatoes cooling down. They taste good and keep life interesting, too! Serve this as a side dish – it goes particularly well with grilled salmon and a large green salad.

750g small potatoes (new potatoes or other speciality
    potatoes)
100ml organic kefir (you can use cow's milk kefir, though
    I've found home-made goat's milk kefir tastes
    particularly tangy – see page 180)
1 Scotch bonnet yellow chilli pepper
1 garlic clove, peeled and chopped
A small handful of fresh coriander, chopped

If using new potatoes such as Jersey Royals, wash or scrub them well and leave the skins on. If using speciality purple potatoes, which have thicker skins, quickly peel the skins.

Boil the potatoes until soft in the middle but not too soft – you want them to hold firm when you slice them.

Drain the cooked potatoes, then rinse them under cold running water to cool down.

While the potatoes are cooling, make the dressing. Put the kefir, Scotch bonnet, garlic, coriander and salt in a blender and pulse until smooth.

Pour the sauce over the potatoes and let the flavours soak in.

Serve cold.

WATERCRESS, ORANGE and ① ②
BEETROOT ONE-BOWL SALAD

This is a 5-minute lunch. Serve it with cold smoked mackerel or poached salmon on the side, ready-cooked from the supermarket.

1 bag of watercress
1 orange, peeled and chopped
4 beetroots, chopped
3 tbsp olive oil
1 tbsp apple cider vinegar
1 tsp English mustard powder

Assemble the plants in a serving bowl.

Mix the oil, vinegar and mustard in a cup, then pour over the other ingredients and serve immediately.

CURLY CUCUMBER ①②
and SAUERKRAUT SALAD

Serves 2

This contains probiotic sauerkraut, to plant beneficial bacteria in the gut.

½ cucumber, spiralized into ribbons
12 radishes, sliced
2 large forkfuls of sauerkraut (fermented cabbage)
2 tbsp virgin olive oil
Juice of ½ lemon
1 tsp English mustard powder
Sea salt and freshly ground black pepper, to taste

Assemble the first three ingredients in a bowl.

In a cup, stir together the olive oil, lemon juice and mustard powder.

Pour the dressing over the salad. Season, then serve immediately.

FIVE (ALMOST) NAKED INSTANT SIDE DISHES

1. Empty a bag of lamb's lettuce into a bowl, then drizzle over extra virgin olive oil and balsamic vinegar to your liking.

2. Buy a radicchio lettuce, wash and chop it finely, squeeze over the juice of an orange and drizzle extra virgin olive oil on top. Add a handful of walnuts and a little sea salt and pepper.

3. Top and tail a fennel bulb, then cut it into slivers, drizzle over the juice of one lemon and some extra virgin olive oil and season with some sea salt and ground black pepper.

4. Slice two ripe tomatoes, drizzle with extra virgin olive oil and balsamic vinegar and mix with a few Kalamata olives.

5. Slice half a cucumber, take a small matchbox-size piece of Roquefort and crumble it over, then add the juice of a squeezed lemon and a drizzle of virgin olive oil.

Protein

PIL PIL PRAWNS with GREEN LEAVES ①②

Serves 2

This Spanish dish can be knocked up in ten minutes, so it's great for after work or as a quick lunch – simply throw the prawns over the top of a large pile of green leaves. Use whatever takes your fancy – from rocket or lamb's lettuce to sorrel or purslane. Cruise your supermarket shelves, or the stalls at a farmers' market, and choose some green leaves out of your normal comfort zone so you get some diversity into your diet to feed your gut flora.

3 tbsp extra virgin olive oil
3 garlic cloves, peeled and finely chopped
1 small chilli, finely chopped
240g peeled prawns (either raw or cooked)
A sprinkling of paprika
Juice of 1 lemon
A small handful of fresh flat-leaf parsley, finely chopped
Sea salt and freshly ground black pepper, to taste

To serve:
A pile of green leaves drizzled in a little extra virgin olive
   oil and a squeeze of lemon

Gently heat the oil in a frying pan then add the garlic and chilli and let it sizzle for a couple of minutes. While the garlic is still white (not turned golden), add the prawns and stir until coated. If using raw prawns, wait for them to turn from grey to pink in colour.

Add the paprika, lemon juice and the parsley and stir round. Season to taste.

Place a pile of dressed green leaves on each serving plate, then throw your prawns on top and serve.

SEA BASS with PRESERVED LEMONS ①②

Serves 2

This is very quick and easy – about 15 minutes from start to finish. It goes well with the harissa potato salad (page 143), the cooked carrot and coriander salad (page 141) and the kefir courgettes (page 142).

3 tbsp extra virgin olive oil
½ red onion, finely chopped
1 tomato, chopped
2 preserved lemons (also sometimes known as pickled lemons)
A handful of fresh flat-leaf parsley, chopped
2 sea bass fillets
A pinch of sea salt
A sprinkling of sumac

Heat 2 tablespoons of the olive oil in a frying pan on a medium heat, then add the onion and cook for about 5 minutes.

Add the tomato and lemons and sizzle for about 5 minutes on a low heat.

Add the flat-leaf parsley.

Pat the sea bass fillets dry with some kitchen paper and sprinkle a little salt and sumac onto each one.

Sweep the lemon/tomato mixture to one side of the pan and add the remaining tablespoon of olive oil to the other side of the pan. Cook the fish there for about 5 minutes, turning to cook on each side. If the fillet is thin, it should change colour from transparent to white quite quickly. Be careful not to overcook the fish, otherwise it could go dry.

Transfer the cooked fish to serving plates and top with the glossy tomato/lemon mixture.

ALMOND and ①② CAULIFLOWER PASANDA

Serves 4

This is a one-bowl meal. I'm using swede here to replace white potato, which often goes nicely with cauliflower in curries. Swedes are cheap and delicious, and very much a forgotten vegetable that's good to get into your repertoire, for added variety.

3 tbsp coconut oil

1 onion, finely chopped

3cm fresh ginger, peeled and finely grated

2 garlic cloves, peeled and finely chopped

1 small chilli, deseeded and chopped

¼ tsp garam masala

1 tsp ground cumin

2 tsp ground coriander

1 tsp turmeric powder

½ tsp chilli powder (optional)

1 swede, peeled and cubed

1 cauliflower, central stem cut out and broken into
   florets

1 large carrot, peeled and cubed

400ml water

300g ground almonds

160ml coconut cream

Sea salt, to taste

To serve:

A handful of pomegranate seeds

Juice of ½ lime

A handful of fresh coriander, chopped

Melt the coconut oil in a pan on a medium heat and
add the onion, ginger, garlic and chopped chilli and stir
around. Let them sweat and go a little transparent, then

add the garam masala, cumin and coriander and, if using, a little chilli powder.

Add all the vegetables and stir until they are coated with the curry mixture.

Add the water and salt, then lower the heat and let the curry simmer for about 30 minutes or until the vegetables are cooked through and tender.

Stir in the ground almonds and the coconut cream then serve garnished with pomegranate seeds, a squeeze of fresh lime and a sprinkling of fresh coriander.

ROSEMARY and ORANGE ①② ROAST CHICKEN

Serves 4

1 whole chicken
1 orange
3 tbsp extra virgin olive oil
A few sprigs of fresh rosemary
Sea salt and freshly ground black pepper, to taste

Heat the oven to 160°C.

Put the chicken in a roasting tin. Cut the orange in half, then squeeze the juice from one half over the chicken and put the orange half inside the chicken with the other unsqueezed half. The orange's flavour and juice will ooze from the cavity into the meat and prevent it getting dry.

Scrunch up the rosemary sprigs and stuff them inside the bird with the orange. Drizzle the olive oil over the chicken and season, then roast in the oven for 2 hours so the bird cooks long and slow. The meat should be falling off the bone when you take it out of the oven. To test the chicken to see if it is done, pierce the thigh with the tip of a sharp knife and if the juices run clear, the chicken is cooked. When the chicken is ready, remove it from the oven and leave it to rest for 10 minutes, covered with a piece of tin foil.

Once the chicken has rested, cut the breast into slices, remove the legs and wings and divide them among your diners with a serving of the nice crispy skin for each person.

Scrape the juices from the pan and drizzle them over each portion.

Retrieve all the bones after the meal for making your own home-made chicken stock.

GRILLED SALMON with GINGER DRESSING ①②

Serves 4

For many years I didn't take any notice of the grill setting on my oven. I wasn't quite sure how to use it, and presumed it would be messy and smelly. Then I read a couple of nice recipes which involved a grill and decided to dig out the oven instructions and find out how to use the grill bit. It was so worth the effort. A couple of minutes and a very obvious setting on the dial later, I now grill fish regularly – it gives it such a lovely flavour and keeps the fish moist inside whilst crisping it slightly on the outside. If you haven't discovered your grill setting, do try it, you may not look back. This recipe has been adapted from *Leith's Fish Bible*. This goes well alongside a mountain of Asian stir-fried vegetables and can be served hot or cold, so it is ideal for packed lunches and leftover meals, too.

4 salmon fillets (if you want to avoid bones, choose the
   tail ends)
A drizzle of virgin olive oil
Sea salt and freshly ground black pepper, to taste

For the dressing:
2 tbsp rice wine vinegar
4 tbsp extra virgin olive oil
2 tbsp tamari
2 spring onions
1 tbsp maple syrup
2cm fresh ginger, peeled and grated
2 tbsp chopped fresh coriander

Put the salmon, drizzled in a little olive oil and seasoned, under the grill on a high setting and cook either side until cooked through (you can test with a knife to see if it is firm).

Meanwhile, make the dressing – put all the ingredients in a small bowl and mix together.

To serve, put a salmon fillet on each plate and drizzle with some of the dressing.

GRILLED SALMON with CLOUDY ①② LEMON JUICE and PARSLEY

Serves 4

This is a favourite based on a version I first saw in one of Gwyneth Paltrow's recipe books. If you cook a large piece like this, it often gives good leftovers. This is lovely with roast parsnip and carrot chips (page 132) or sticky Jerusalem artichokes (page 135).

850g piece of salmon fillet
150ml extra virgin olive oil, plus extra for drizzling
2 unwaxed lemons
A small bunch of fresh flat-leaf parsley, chopped
Sea salt and freshly ground black pepper, to taste

Place the salmon on a baking sheet, drizzle with a little olive oil and season.

Cut the lemons in half and place them cut-side down on the sheet around the edges of the salmon.

Place the sheet under the grill set to a medium heat and cook the salmon and lemons for 8–10 minutes until it looks done. The time needed will depend on the thickness of the salmon. I don't usually need to turn the fish over to get it cooked through – you want to be able to prod it with a knife so it's still moist in the middle, and not dried out.

Take the salmon out of the grill. Pick up the lemons with a tea towel (they may be rather hot to handle) and squeeze the juice from them in a lemon squeezer, making sure the pips are strained out. Transfer the juice to a small bowl.

Add the 150ml of olive oil to the squeezed cloudy lemon juice, and add a little sea salt and the chopped parsley.

Cut the fish into portions and serve on each plate with a spoonful of the dressing on top.

CHICKEN NUGGETS ①②

Serves 4–6

A hit with the whole family, these taste delicious both hot or at room temperature as leftovers the next day. Try them with spiralized sweet potatoes and wilted spinach.

200g ground almonds
1 tsp English mustard powder
2 tbsp arrowroot
1 tsp paprika

½ tsp cayenne pepper

1 tsp sea salt

120ml extra virgin olive oil

700g chicken breast cut into mini fillets (about 16–20)

Heat the oven to 220°C.

Combine the ground almonds, mustard powder, arrowroot, paprika, cayenne pepper and salt in a bowl.

Pour the olive oil into another bowl.

Take each mini fillet and dip it in the oil, then roll it around in the powder mixture and place each one alongside each other in a baking dish.

Bake in the oven for about 20 minutes until the nuggets are golden brown.

SLOW-COOKED PORK ①②
and APPLE STEW

Serves 4

I've been cooking this in different guises for years – it makes the house smell of comfort cooking. The meat should be easy to digest because of the long cooking time, and stewed apples contain pectin, a prebiotic fibre that helps feed the good bacteria in your gut. Serve with a side dish of roast vegetables, sauerkraut or stir-fried red cabbage, or just with a simple bowl of steamed carrots drizzled with virgin olive oil.

6 tbsp extra virgin olive oil

800g pork loin, cubed

2 red onions, cut into eighths

3 apples, peeled and grated

½ teaspoon dried thyme, or a few stalks of fresh thyme

250ml fresh bone stock (see page 184)

250ml water

60ml apple cider vinegar

Sea salt and freshly ground black pepper, to taste

Heat the oven to 160°C.

Heat 3 tablespoons of olive oil in a casserole and cook the meat on all sides until the raw pink colour has disappeared.

Remove the meat and juices to a bowl to rest while you cook the onions in the casserole with the remaining 3 tablespoons of olive oil until translucent and sweating.

Add the grated apples to the onions and mix through, then stir in the thyme, stock, water and apple cider vinegar.

Transfer the casserole to the oven with the lid on and cook for at least 3 hours. Check from time to time to make sure the sauce isn't too thick; if it is, add a little more water. Alternatively, cook in a pressure cooker following the manufacturer's instructions.

When cooked, season to taste and serve in a bowl (you may find it easier to eat with a spoon!).

SLOW-COOKED LAMB   ①②
and SPINACH CURRY

Serves 4–5

This curry is an anti-inflammatory powerhouse and a great support for any inflammatory condition. Turmeric, ginger, coconut oil and coriander all have anti-inflammatory properties. If you use organic lamb, there is likely to be more omega-3 essential fatty acids than in intensively reared meat, and omega-3 is another anti-inflammatory. The chicken stock is included for a healthy gut lining. This dish makes marvellous leftovers and freezes well, too.

3 tbsp coconut oil

1kg lamb fillet, diced

2 red onions, cut into eighths

1–2 chilli peppers, deseeded and finely chopped

2cm fresh ginger, peeled and grated

1 tsp garam masala

1 tsp ground turmeric

1 tsp ground cumin

2 x 400g tins whole plum tomatoes

160ml tin coconut cream

240ml fresh chicken stock (page 184)

260g bag of spinach leaves, washed

½ tsp sea salt

A handful of fresh coriander, chopped, to serve

Heat 1 tablespoon of the oil in a pan on a medium heat, add the meat and cook, turning, until it is no longer pink.

In a separate pan, add the remaining 2 tablespoons of oil and melt on a medium heat. Add the onions, chillies and all the spices and sauté for about 5 minutes until the onions are soft. Tip in the tomatoes and stir through.

Transfer the tomato and vegetable spice mixture to the meat pan, then put on a lid and gently simmer for about 3 hours on a low heat. Alternatively, put the mixture in a casserole dish with a lid on in the oven at 160°C for about 3 hours. Check the curry from time to time; if the mixture looks too thick, add a few drops of water.

When the meat is tender and soft and has taken on a deep red, glossy hue, remove the pan from the heat and add a teaspoon of sea salt. Add a handful of spinach to the curry at a time, and stir until all the leaves have wilted. The curry should be piping hot from the oven, so the spinach should wilt easily. I like to do it this way, rather than over the hob, otherwise the spinach can become overcooked, stringy and tasteless.

Serve with a cauliflower which has been finely shredded and sautéed in a little coconut oil. (You can buy these ready chopped in many supermarkets if you need to save time.)

ASIAN CHICKEN CUCUMBER SALAD ①②

Serves 2

This works equally nicely when you replace the chicken with cooked prawns.

300g cooked chicken (e.g. leftovers from a roast), sliced
2 large carrots, peeled and cut into matchsticks
1 cucumber, spiralized
½ small red onion, sliced into fine half moons
A handful of fresh coriander, chopped
40g salted roasted peanuts

Dressing:
Juice of 1 lime
2 tbsp fish sauce
A sprinkling of dried chilli flakes, to taste
1 tsp raw honey
1 garlic clove, peeled and chopped
2 tbsp virgin olive oil

Assemble the chicken, carrots and cucumber on a large serving plate.

Sprinkle over the red onion, coriander and roasted peanuts.

Mix all the ingredients for the dressing together in a cup and pour over the salad and serve immediately.

TRAY-BAKED CHICKEN ①②
with OLIVES and SAGE

Serves 4

This dish takes just minutes to prepare and produces a delicious dinner and great leftovers for packed lunches. While you are waiting for the chicken to cook, you could be tucking into a grapefruit starter to take the edge off your hunger, prime your digestive system for the main meal and clock up another plant portion. This goes well with a side of roasted potatoes (just take your cold potatoes out of the fridge, drizzle in extra virgin olive oil and sea salt and a handful of fresh chopped rosemary, if you have some) and a side mountain of rocket leaves drizzled in a little extra virgin olive oil and balsamic vinegar.

1kg chicken thighs and/or drumsticks
3 tbsp extra virgin olive oil
A handful of fresh sage leaves (about 30g), chopped
150g pitted Kalamata olives
4 garlic cloves, peeled and crushed with the back of a
   knife
1 tsp sea salt
Freshly ground black pepper, to taste

Heat the oven to 200°C.

Put the chicken in an oven dish, drizzle over the olive oil, sprinkle over the chopped sage, olives, garlic and seasoning and roast for 40 minutes, turning the chicken halfway through the cooking time.

Remove from the oven when the chicken is crispy and cooked through. Test it to see if it is done; pierce the thigh with the tip of a sharp knife and if the juices run clear, the chicken is cooked. Remove the cooked chicken from the oven and leave it to rest for 15 minutes, covered with a piece of tin foil then slice and serve.

SIRLOIN STEAK with ROCKET ①② and BALSAMIC

Serves 2

The most absorbable form of iron comes from red meat, so including a steak in your diet once a week can help your energy levels. The vitamin C contained in green leaves such as rocket can help absorption of the iron, so the ingredients here make a good combination. People sometimes worry that red meat may lead to cancer, however, big studies on red meat consumption that I have seen haven't measured how many vegetables the subjects were eating. High vegetable consumption, as we know, reduces the risk of cancer. Also, the quality of the red meat isn't usually described, and when the studies are done on large groups of North Americans, you can bet the meat being eaten isn't organic (therefore more likely to contain residues of antibiotics) and they aren't eating seven plants a day! Twenty or thirty years ago, obtaining an organic steak wasn't easy. Now, most large supermarkets offer them, so access is much easier than it used to be. In my opinion, red meat is all about quality, rather than quantity.

2 x 200g steaks – the best-quality you can afford,
    preferably organic
2 tbsp extra virgin olive oil
Coarse sea salt, e.g. Maldon, for sprinkling
A bag of rocket leaves
Balsamic vinegar, to drizzle

Heat 1 tablespoon of olive oil in a frying pan and cook the steaks for 6–8 minutes on each side.

Remove the steaks from the pan, set on cutting board and sprinkle with coarse sea salt.

Divide the rocket amongst each plate and drizzle with the remaining olive oil and the balsamic vinegar.

Place the steaks on top and serve. Chew well!

CRISPY SHEPHERD'S PIE ①②

Serves 4

8 tbsp extra virgin olive oil

1 onion, finely chopped

1 celery stick, finely chopped

2 garlic cloves, peeled and finely chopped

500g minced beef

400ml home-made chicken stock or other bone broth
  (page 184)

2 tsp sea salt

1 tbsp apple cider vinegar

1 tbsp tomato purée

2 medium sweet potatoes (one orange variety, one white
  variety, if you wish)

Pour 4 tablespoons of olive oil into a large saucepan on a medium heat, add the onion, celery and garlic and sauté for about 5 minutes until they become translucent. Add the beef and stir into the mixture until it is no longer pink. Pour in the stock or broth, then stir in 1 teaspoon of salt, the vinegar and tomato purée. Simmer on a low heat for about an hour (or longer if you have a slow cooker, and more time) to get the meat really tender and digestible.

Meanwhile, peel the potatoes and spiralize them on the setting that produces long, flat, thin ribbons. Put the ribbons in a large bowl and mix with the remaining 4 tablespoons of olive oil and add a teaspoon of sea salt. Thoroughly mix the oil in with the ribbons – you can toss these around with your hands or a wooden spoon.

Heat the oven to 230°C.

When the meat mixture is cooked, pour it into a baking dish. Spread the potato ribbons on top, to cover all the meat. Put the pie in the oven and bake for about 25 minutes or until the top is crispy, then serve alongside some steamed green vegetables or broccoli.

REAL SPANISH TORTILLA   ①②

Serves 4

This meal uses the simplest ingredients and is all about technique and having the right kit. Once you've made this once, you can reproduce this to eternity. It's a brilliant meal that tastes good and is very portable, so perfect for packed lunches. The reason why this recipe is in this book is that it is usually eaten at room temperature when it has cooled down, or cold the next day – hence it is a meal full of resistant starch which contain those prebiotic fibres to feed the good bacteria in your gut.

People sometimes think Spanish tortilla will be oily, but if you do it right it shouldn't be – the olive oil is drained off but leaves its delicious flavour behind.

500ml extra virgin olive oil, plus 4 tbsp for cooking

800g peeled potatoes, roughly chopped to discs a similar
    size and thickness

1 onion, roughly chopped into chunks of similar size to
    the potato

2 eggs

2 tsp sea salt

Heat the 500ml oil in a large frying pan on a medium
heat and cook the potatoes and onions. The oil should
not be boiling, just gently simmering. You want the potatoes and onions to cook through until moist, without
going brown.

Stir the potatoes every so often, checking they are
all covered in the oil. This is my top tip, learnt from
my teenage Spanish exchange partner Mari Carmen's
mother, Carmen, for an authentic Spanish omelette:
prod the potatoes with a fork so they break up in the oil.
Gently here and there, prod and prod. You're aiming for
the potatoes to get a little more surface area.

When the potatoes aren't brown but are falling apart
if you prod them with your fork, switch off the heat and,
with a slotted spoon, gently scoop the potatoes out of the
oil into a colander or sieve set above a big bowl to catch
the olive oil. You may want to dab the potatoes with
some kitchen paper, to soak up some of the oil.

Meanwhile, tip the olive oil left in the pan into a bowl
to be disposed of. Don't reuse oil that has been used for

frying as when it is refried it can form trans fats, which are dangerous to heart and brain health.

Now whisk the eggs in a separate large bowl and fold in the cooked potatoes and onion. Season with salt.

Heat 2 tablespoons of olive oil in the pan, add the eggy mixture and cook for about 15 minutes on a low heat. Go slow and wait for the mixture to start to set around the edges and you can slightly smell the bottom of the egg mixture browning.

Take a spatula and ease the set egg away from the sides of the pan. Put a large dinner plate over the top of the pan and turn the pan upside down so the omelette can fall into the plate. Then put 2 tablespoons of olive oil into the pan and slide the omelette back in to cook the other side on a low heat for a few short minutes. This side usually cooks much quicker than the other, just a few minutes.

Slide the omelette out of the pan onto a clean dinner plate with a piece of kitchen paper on it and wait for the omelette to cool down. Cut the omelette into four and serve cold.

Serve with a portion of warm paprika tomatoes (page 137) and a few green olives stuffed with anchovies on the side.

DUCK RED THAI CURRY   ①②

Serves 4

When buying a red curry paste, read the label well, check there is no gluten in it and that the ingredients are all real food that you can understand. There are some *Gut Makeover*-friendly unprocessed ones out there without additives and preservatives, if you look. This dish tastes great reheated the next day as a leftover lunch and freezes well, too. The curry goes well with a side dish of stir-fried tat soi, morning glory, or pak choi – all can be found in the Asian section of supermarket vegetable departments.

2 tbsp coconut oil

2 pear shallots or a small onion, chopped

1 tbsp Thai red curry paste

2 duck breasts, cut into thin strips (up to you if you keep some of the fat on)

½ head of cauliflower, broken into small florets

1 red bell pepper, deseeded and cut into thin strips

8 organic mushrooms

400ml tin coconut milk

2 tbsp fish sauce

1 tbsp tamari sauce

Juice of 1 lime

Melt the coconut oil in a large pan on a medium heat. Add the shallots or onion and stir round to coat in the oil.

Add the Thai red curry paste, stir it into the shallot/onion and cook for a minute or two and then, when it is hot, add the duck and stir from time to time. When the duck is cooked through and is no longer pink, add the vegetables and stir together so they are coated with the curry paste.

Pour in the coconut milk and cook on a medium heat, then let the mixture simmer for 10–15 minutes, until the cauliflower is cooked through and just tender – don't let it go too soft, you don't want your vegetables mushy!

Add the fish sauce, tamari and lime juice and serve at once.

COD with SAGE   ①②

Serves 4

This is an absolute favourite of mine, and terribly simple and quick to make after work.

4 x 150g pieces of cod
4 tbsp extra virgin olive oil or 2 tbsp oil and a large knob
   of butter (Phase 2)
A bunch of fresh sage, finely chopped
Sea salt and freshly ground black pepper, to taste

Dab the fish pieces with a piece of kitchen paper so it isn't wet, then season with salt and pepper.

Pour the oil/butter into a pan and heat on a medium flame, then add the fish and the sage.

Cook for about 5 minutes on one side then turn (the length of time will depend on the thickness of the fish, but you can prod it with a fork and see if it flakes away to see if it is ready).

When cooked, serve with a little of the herby juice from the pan and a couple of sides of fresh vegetables of your choice. (Roast fennel and roast tomatoes go particularly well with this.)

GERMAN MARINATED ①② SLOW-COOKED POT BEEF

Serves 4–6

This is one of my favourite German mother-in-law dishes. I remember the first time Hildegard and her husband came to stay with my husband and I in London, she flew over from Cologne with this dish in a Tupperware pot for our dinner. I'd never met anyone who had done that before, but I was delighted to be the recipient sharing that meal. It just needed a gentle reheat in its own juices and a few vegetable sides. This is the kind of protein meal you could cook at the weekend to use for a big family meal, and have leftovers to put in packed lunches and stir-fries in the days afterwards.

1 onion, chopped

1 large carrot, peeled and cubed

250ml red wine vinegar

500ml water

1 tsp mixed spice

1 tsp ground white peppercorns

1 bay leaf

1 tsp juniper berries (if you can find them)

1kg piece of beef topside (you could use beef brisket,
which is cheaper, but needs longer marinating and
cooking time)

2 tbsp extra virgin olive oil

2 tbsp honey

1 tbsp cornflour

Sea salt and freshly ground black pepper, to taste

Place the onion and carrot in a pan with the red wine vinegar and water. Add the mixed spice, white peppercorns, bay leaf and, if you are using them, juniper berries and bring to the boil. Let this cool down.

Add the beef to the cooled mixture and leave to marinate in the fridge overnight or, if you have more time, up to three days. The cheaper the cut of meat, the longer you'll need to marinate it to tenderize it.

Take the beef out of the marinade, pat dry with kitchen paper and season with sea salt and a little black pepper.

Put the olive oil in a pan and heat over a medium

flame, then add the beef and roll it around, gently cooking for about 5 minutes to brown it a little.

Add the marinade mixture to the beef and bring to the boil, then simmer on a gentle heat for at least 2–3 hours. Alternatively, cook it in a pressure cooker or a slow cooker, following the manufacturer's instructions. You want the meat to come out extremely tender and slightly falling apart.

At the end, use a whisk to stir the honey and cornflour into the juices.

Remove the beef from the cooking liquid, cut it into slices and place them in a large serving bowl with a few ladles of the juice on top. Serve with a selection of side vegetables, such as roasted mixed veg and mashed swede.

ASIAN ROASTED CRISPY PORK BELLY ①②

Serves 4

This is a recipe adapted from one by Gok Wan. Pork belly is a very fatty meat and *The Gut Makeover* is moderate on the fat front, encouraging you to use the amount you need for cooking and to make food taste good, rather than going mad with it. However, we do need a certain amount of saturated fats, preferably from animal fats, to make sex hormones (libido!) and so that our brains function well. So, especially if you can't eat butter or Roquefort (good sources of animal fats) due to an intolerance on the dairy front, this might be a good recipe to use now and again to get the benefits from some quality saturated fat. Make sure you chew really thoroughly for good digestion and absorption.

It's super delicious and makes great leftovers – it works well both transported and eaten at room temperature in packed lunches the next day, or sliced thinly into stir-fries the day after.

800g piece of pork belly
1 tbsp rice vinegar
Juice of 1 lemon
2 tsp Chinese five-spice powder
1 tsp ground white pepper
2 tsp sea salt

Gently slice off the top layer of fat on the pork belly – this is the rind-looking layer which can be very tough, so I cut this off then crisscross the softer fat that remains underneath. Then turn it over and score the meat side with crisscrosses from side to side. Doing this on both sides will provide entry points for the spices in the meat and vinegar/lemon to tenderize the fat on top.

Put the meat in a roasting tin and rub the vinegar and lemon juice on the fat side, then turn over. Now rub the five-spice powder, white pepper and half of the salt into the meat side. Put the tin in the fridge overnight to marinate.

Take the meat out of the fridge a couple of hours before cooking to come to room temperature.

Heat the oven to 160°C.

Roast the meat for 40 minutes, with the meat side facing up, then turn over and increase the oven temperature to 220°C and cook for 20 minutes until the fat side is crisp, brown and the texture of pork scratchings.

Take out of the oven, cover with tin foil and let the meat rest for 20 minutes before cutting into thin slices and serving.

CRISPY REHEATED POTATOES ①② with POACHED EGGS

Cook a batch of jacket potatoes in your oven, then leave them out to cool and store them in your fridge for a few days. They will come in handy for chopping into salads, or to slice and gently pan-fry in a little extra virgin olive oil until they go golden and the skins crisp up.

3 tbsp extra virgin olive oil

1 cooked, then cooled, jacket potato

1 red onion, thinly sliced

A sprinkling of cayenne pepper and paprika, to taste

Large handful of spinach, washed

2 eggs

1 tbsp vinegar

Sprinkling of sea salt

Heat the olive oil in a frying pan on a medium heat, then gently sauté the potato and onion.

Sprinkle the pepper and paprika on top and leave to cook for 5–10 minutes, turning the potato over from time to time until it is crispy on both sides.

Add the spinach and stir until it has wilted (usually a couple of minutes).

Make poached eggs using vinegar and following the recipe on page 71.

Pile the potato, onion and spinach mixture onto a plate and slide your poached eggs on top, sprinkled with a little sea salt.

SPINACH and ROQUEFORT 'PANCAKES' ②

Serves 1

3 knobs of butter
2 eggs, beaten
200g spinach leaves, washed
Small matchbox-size piece of Roquefort cheese
Sea salt and freshly ground black pepper, to taste

Melt one knob of butter in a non-stick frying pan. Add half the beaten eggs and swirl around the pan until it is completely covered and you have a thin pancake-looking shape filling the space of the pan. On a medium heat, let the egg start to set and then flip over and cook the other side.

Repeat the exercise again with another knob of butter and the remaining egg.

Put the two 'pancakes' on a plate to one side.

In a separate pan, melt the remaining butter, then add the spinach and cook on a medium heat until wilted – this should take less than 5 minutes. Sprinkle over a little sea salt and a good grinding of black pepper.

Place half the spinach on one side of each pancake, then crumble the Roquefort cheese over the two pancakes. Fold over each pancake to enclose the filling and serve.

Stocks, kefirs and tea masterclass

Making kefir

Making kefir is easy. This is my bulletproof version, which should come out like a thick drinking yoghurt with a slightly tart taste, or even a little bit fizzy. Home-made kefir will keep for 2–4 weeks in the fridge.

Equipment:
A plastic sieve (must not be metal)
A wooden spoon (do not use metal cutlery)
A 1-litre Mason jar
A cloth
An elastic band

How to make cow's milk kefir ②

Use organic, non-homogenised milk here; choosing organic means there is less chance of antibiotic residues that could hamper the growth of bacteria in your kefir, while non-homogenised, in my experience, has a better success rate with nice, thick consistency. Duchy Originals milk at Waitrose is non-homogenised. You can buy kefir grains online – they look like white wet sponges and in my experience work better than freeze-dried versions.

500ml organic non-homogenised whole milk
250ml organic single cream
1 tbsp kefir grains

Take the milk and cream out of the fridge for a couple of hours before you make this kefir – they ideally need to be at room temperature before you start work.

Pour the milk and cream into a Mason jar, add the kefir grains and stir with a wooden or plastic spoon.

Put a cloth over the top of the Mason jar, secure it with an elastic band and leave the kefir for up to 48 hours, at room temperature, to ferment. You can remove the cloth and stir it from time to time if you like – once or twice a day.

When the kefir has set, stir it, and strain out the kefir grains using a non-metallic sieve. Transfer to a clean Mason jar and store the kefir in the fridge.

Take the used kefir grains, rinse them and store them in a pot of water in the fridge for a few days until you need to use them for another batch.

Over time the kefir grains grow and get bigger. You can break off sections and give them to friends to start making their own kefir or, if the lump gets too big, break off bits and throw them away. You only need about a tablespoon of grains per batch, otherwise the kefir can become the extreme end of sour and it won't be palatable.

How to make goat's milk kefir ②

I'm currently sourcing unhomogenised raw goat's milk from a local farmer's market. Raw milk, if you can get hold of it, has more bacteria in it than pasteurised milk, where much of the bacteria has been stripped out, so raw milk means bigger billions of bacteria in your kefir.

Goat's milk kefir isn't my cuppa in a breakfast shake – it tastes too much like goat's cheese, which I personally don't like mixed with fruit (you may be OK with it, if so, go for it). However, I find goat's milk kefir tastes delicious in salad dressings where you want a bit of a goat's cheese twang, knowing there are billions of useful bacteria (if buying just regular goat's cheese in a supermarket, one has no idea how long it has been fermented for, and if it has any chance of delivering big bacterial numbers).

Individuals who are lactose intolerant can often tolerate kefir OK because the lactose has been pre-digested by the fermentation process (but not always – so try it out for yourself). However, some can't tolerate it because they are reacting to certain proteins in the milk (rather than the milk sugars, the lactose). If you suspect this is the case, it may well be worth trying goat's milk kefir instead, as it delivers a different set of proteins to cow's milk, and you may find goat's milk has a set of proteins you are OK with.

500ml raw unhomogenised goat's milk
1 tbsp kefir grains

Pour the goat's milk into the Mason jar and add the kefir grains, stirring them with a plastic or wooden spoon. Put a cloth over the top of the Mason jar and secure it with an elastic band.

Place the jar somewhere warm in the house, e.g. an airing cabinet, or a room which is cosy and warm (as opposed to a cold kitchen) and leave for around 48 hours, stirring from time to time with your plastic or wooden spoon.

When it has begun to set, sift out the grains, wash them and place in your fridge in a plastic pot until needed again (as for cow's milk kefir).

Pour the kefir into a clean Mason jar and store in your fridge until needed.

How to make coconut kefir   ②

Although many people who are lactose intolerant do manage to tolerate kefir because the lactose is already broken down by the fermentation process, if you are reacting to the proteins in the milk (e.g. casein, whey, etc.) then dairy kefirs are not going to work for you, and coconut kefir may be a good alternative. Coconut versions are available in health-food stores but are pricey, so if this is something you're planning to have habitually, it's well worth making it yourself. It is very rich, so it's best used as a dessert – e.g. a large dollop with a piece of chopped-up fruit each day.

400ml tin coconut milk
1 tbsp kefir grains

Follow all the instructions as per the goat's milk kefir overleaf. Important note: when it has begun to set, or looks slightly effervescent, you will know it is time to sieve out the grains, wash them and place in the fridge.

How to make bone stocks

You may be wondering what the difference is between bone broths and bone stocks? Nothing. I use the term stock because I'm old-fashioned and that's the term I was brought up with.

Stocks cooked from real animal bones are full of collagen, which is useful for building up the strength of your gut lining – either healing a leaky gut or preventing one developing. A leaky gut (impaired intestinal permeability) often goes hand in hand with dysbiosis (an imbalance in gut flora in the colon further down). So if you sort out the leaky gut, often the bloating further down begins to correct itself. It also contains electrolytes – these are micro minerals such as potassium, magnesium and calcium, which you could become low in, if you are someone who regularly suffers loose stools. Boosting your micro-minerals, if you are regularly losing them, could really help improve your energy levels and mood. Adding this as a base to your soups, stews, stir-fries and even potato salad (mixed with a vinaigrette) could really up the gut-supporting nutritional content of your diet.

There should be no mystery around bone stocks – they are simply a self-assembly job. There can be something very therapeutic about making stock, the gentle bubbling of the bones simmering away, creating a powerhouse of nutritional goodness for you. It's about establishing the habit of making them – say at the beginning of the month – and loading up your freezer with small plastic containers of stock to whip out at every opportunity. Once you've done this, you may never use a stock cube again.

REAL CHICKEN STOCK   ①②

Makes at least 1 litre

1 chicken carcass and bones, meat picked off
1 litre filtered water
1 celery stick, washed
1 carrot, washed, topped and tailed
1 onion, peeled
2 bay leaves

Put the chicken carcass and bones in a large saucepan and add enough of the water to completely cover the chicken, but do not fill the pan too much or the stock may turn out too watery. Add the celery, carrot, onion and bay leaves.

Bring to the boil, then simmer with the lid on for 3–4 hours, or cook it for half an hour in a pressure cooker. Leave the stock to cool, then pour it through a sieve and discard the bones and vegetables. Pour the clear stock into several containers (I usually divide into four or five plastic containers' worth from the bones of one chicken).

You can keep the stock in the fridge for 4–5 days or freeze it and defrost when needed. If you like, you can pour the stock into an ice-cube tray to give you smaller portions that you can pop out, a few at a time, when needed to go into soups, stir-fries and potato salads.

LAMB or BEEF STOCK   ①②

You can often pick up large bags of bones from butchers' shops – just ask. If you're a regular customer, butchers often give them for free, or charge a minimal fee such as a pound or two.

A big bag of lamb or beef bones
3 bay leaves
1 carrot, unpeeled
1 onion, cut in half
1 celery stick

Heat the oven to 180°C.

Place the bones on a baking tray and cook in the oven for 20–30 minutes so they no longer have a pink-round-the-edges, raw look about them. I do this because I find roasting them gives the stock a richer flavour.

Put the bones in a large saucepan, pressure cooker or slow cooker and fill with water until the bones are covered.* Add the bay leaves, carrot, onion and celery and bring to the boil, then lower the heat and simmer with a lid on for as many hours as you can stand.

When you've all had enough, pour the stock through a sieve into a large container and wait for it to cool down. If some hard fat forms on the top, you could skim this off. Decant the golden stock into smaller containers and place them in the freezer, or keep it in your fridge, where they usually last up to a week on the coolest shelf. Just spoon out into your cooking as needed.

*Note: If using a pressure cooker you could bring it to high pressure in the first few minutes then lower the pressure and cook for 90 minutes. This means little noise and steam in your home. Or follow the instructions on a slow cooker.

HOW TO MAKE REAL GINGER TEA ①②

One of my favourite alternatives to caffeinated drinks like tea and coffee is ginger tea. Pour this into a Thermos flask and Bob's your uncle – a gorgeous, hot, beautiful aromatic drink to sip through the day. The zing of fresh ginger tea can be very energizing; it contains anti-inflammatory compounds and can be soothing to drink.

Large piece of fresh ginger – a big jagged piece the size of
    the palm of your hand
1 litre water

Break up your large piece of fresh ginger and bash each piece with the flat side of a knife till it slightly cracks to release the flavour better (a trick I learned from my Chinese sister-in-law, no less).

Boil the pieces of ginger in water for 30 minutes then strain and pour the liquid into a flask so it is ready for when you want it.

Desserts

COCONUT CHIA and PASSION ①② FRUIT DESSERT

Serves 4

The chia seeds support good digestion by helping to move food along the digestive tract.

400ml tin coconut milk
4 tbsp chia seeds
4 passion fruits

Mix the coconut milk and chia seeds together in a glass bowl and place in the fridge. After 15 minutes, stir the mixture, then after another 15 minutes stir it again to stop the seeds settling at the bottom of the bowl. Leave the mixture to set overnight in the fridge, or for a few hours.

To serve, cut open one passion fruit, scoop out a large spoonful of flesh per person and pop it on top of the chia seed mixture.

CACAO, COCONUT and BLACK ①②
CHERRY CHIA

Serves 4

Cacao nibs – which are raw, bitter real chocolate with absolutely nothing else mixed with them – are bursting with polyphenols, which are plant chemical foods that beneficial bacteria love to graze on. Most chocolates we buy have been mixed with stabilizers, processed oils and, of course, sugar – none of which is much good for us. Hence, if you'd like some chocolate on your *Gut Makeover*, this is the way to do it. The dark colour in the cherries also provides more polyphenols for your gut bacteria.

400ml tin coconut milk
4 tbsp chia seeds
4 tbsp black cherries (buy frozen and defrost if not in season)
4 tbsp roasted flaked almonds
4 tsp cacao nibs

Mix the coconut milk and chia seeds together in a glass bowl and place in the fridge. After 15 minutes, stir the mixture, then after another 15 minutes stir it again to stop the seeds settling at the bottom of the bowl. Leave the mixture to set overnight in the fridge, or for a few hours.

To serve: for each person, take a large spoonful of the chia mix and sprinkle a tablespoon of black cherries and roasted flaked almonds on each portion with a teaspoon of cacao nibs.

CHEESE and GRAPES   ②

Serves 1

Here we have some good bacteria to plant in your gut from the cheese and some polyphenol plant chemicals from the grapes to feed the good bacteria in your gut and help them multiply.

1 small matchbox-size piece of Roquefort cheese, at room
    temperature
A small handful of black or purple grapes

Serve the two ingredients together – I like to spread a bit of cheese onto each grape as I eat them. Forgetting the health benefits, the taste is wonderful.

PAPAYA and LIME JUICE   ①②

Serves 1

You could actually eat this at the start or the end of a meal. The enzymes in the papaya can help break down your forthcoming, or just-eaten meal, for better digestion.

1 small ripe papaya
Juice of ½ lime

Cut the papaya in half, then peel and deseed it.

Place the papaya on a dessert plate and pour over the lime juice.

Sample meal plans

A weekend – Phase 1 or 2

	Saturday	Sunday
Breakfast	Spinach scrambled egg + glass of green gunge	Wild salmon + avocado + glass of green gunge
	Ginger tea	Ginger tea
Lunch	Cup of gazpacho + Fillet of smoked cooked mackerel, cooked beetroot, chicory leaves and French dressing	Roast chicken with lemon and extra virgin olive oil with roasted vegetables + a corn on the cob
Dinner	Bowl of butternut squash/sweet potato soup with roasted walnuts	Mario's orange-onion-olive salad + tin of sardines in olive oil
	Half a mango	Bowl of mushroom soup
Remember at each meal:	Sit down, slow down, chew properly	Sit down, slow down, chew properly

On Saturday, if this plan is executed properly, you should consume at least seven American cup sizes of plants – five as vegetables and two maximum as fruit. I recommend maximum two pieces of fruit or even less, to keep your sugar intake down. Just so you can start to see what this looks like:

On Saturday:

1 cup spinach (in eggs)

1 cup kale, ½ orange, ginger, etc. (in green gunge, a one-person portion)

1 cup beetroot

1 cup chicory

1 cup of gazpacho soup (tomatoes, cucumber, pepper, onion)

1 cup pumpkin/butternut squash

1 cup mango

= 7 and a half cupfuls of plants, six as vegetables and one and a half as fruit.

On Sunday:

1 cup avocado

1 cup kale, ½ orange, ginger, etc. (in green gunge, a one-person portion)

2 cups in roast vegetables, e.g. squash, mushrooms, cauliflower

1 cup sweetcorn

1 orange in the salad

1 cup mushrooms in the soup

= 7 and a half cupfuls of plants, 6 as vegetables, 1 and a half as fruit

You'll see we have covered around 17 different types of vegetables and fruit in this list. We are aiming to eat about 30 different plants a week (the wider the diversity of plants, the wider the diversity of gut flora and the better it is for your health). This weekend plan means we are more than halfway there on variety for the week already.

If you have a large appetite or are of a larger build and need more nutrition, you could even ramp up the plants to another portion or two a day, e.g. you could have 2 cups of squash on Sunday, as they will melt down when baked, and you could add in another cup of pumpkin and have more soup on the Saturday.

A week in Phase 1

Monday	Tuesday	Wednesday	Thursday	Friday	Varieties
Banana nut bread + small green gunge	Ripe sliced avocado + wild salmon + nutty non-dairy breakfast shake	Scrambled eggs + wild salmon + green gunge	Nutty non-dairy shake + spinach eggs	Banana nut bread + small green gunge	Banana Kale Orange Ginger Mint Red onion Courgette Yellow pepper Cherry tomatoes Apple Tomatoes Garlic Rocket Plum Avocado Blueberries Grapefruit Kiwi Beansprouts Broccoli White onion Cabbage Carrots Pear Spring onions Pak choi Lime Cauliflower Turmeric Spinach Melon Strawberries Parsley Olives Nectarine Lemon Radicchio Leeks Sugar snaps
Leftover chicken + roast vegetables	Leftover Bolognese + spiralized courgettes	Gut-healing Asian soup	Lamb and spinach curry + cauliflower rice	Niçoise salad	
Starter: Handful of rocket leaves with balsamic + extra virgin olive oil	Starter: Half a grapefruit	Starter: An avocado with lemon + Tabasco	Starter: A few pieces of chopped pineapple	Starter: Quarter of a radicchio drizzled in extra virgin olive oil + balsamic	
Bolognese + spiralized courgettes	Multi-coloured stir-fry	Lamb and spinach curry + cauliflower 'rice'	Warm green chicken salad	Baked salmon with mustard + almond crust with triple greens	
Piece of fruit	Piece of fruit	Piece of fruit	Piece of fruit	Piece of fruit	
Remember at each meal: Sit down, slow down, chew properly					
7 cups	7 cups	7 cups	7 cups	7 cups	39 varieties

A week in Phase 2, if you can tolerate dairy

Monday	Tuesday	Wednesday	Thursday	Friday
Kefir berry/ banana shake (If you feel this isn't enough to fill you up you could have an egg or salmon dish in the mornings too)	Kefir pine-apple shake	Kefir berry/ banana shake	Kefir pine-apple shake	Kefir berry/ banana shake
Thai organic beef salad	Chicory, pine nut and Roquefort salad	Niçoise salad	Leftover pork schnitzel + potato salad + steamed asparagus	Roast Mediterranean vegetables + omelette
Starter: An avocado with lemon + Tabasco	Starter: Red chicory + orange salad	Starter: Jerusalem artichoke + carrot soup	Starter: Mushroom soup	Starter: Cup of gazpacho
Butternut squash/ sweet potato soup + sautéed chilli walnuts	Pork schnitzel + German potato salad + steamed asparagus	Lebanese lemon chicken livers + watercress	Warm green chicken salad	Peruvian ceviche with red onions, sweet potatoes + corn on the cob
Remember at each meal: Sit down, slow down, chew properly				

A week in Phase 2, if you are non-dairy

Monday	Tuesday	Wednesday	Thursday	Friday
Banana nut bread + small green gunge	Ripe sliced avocado + wild salmon + some cherries or berries with a dollop of coconut kefir	Scrambled eggs + wild salmon + a piece of fruit with a dollop of coconut kefir	Nutty non-dairy shake + a piece of banana nut bread	Banana nut bread + small green gunge
Warm green chicken salad	Chicory + apple salad + walnuts	Leftover pork schnitzel + potato salad + steamed asparagus	Leftover roast vegetables + pumpkin seeds	Leftover chicken livers + pile of watercress with dressing
Starter: A handful of bitter leaves with vinaigrette dressing	Starter: Jerusalem artichoke + carrot soup	Starter: An avocado with lemon + Tabasco	Starter: Radicchio lettuce with balsamic + extra virgin olive oil	Starter: Mushroom soup
Butternut squash/ sweet potato soup + sautéed chilli walnuts	Pork schnitzel + German potato salad + steamed asparagus	Roast mixed vegetables with handful of roasted pumpkin seeds	Lebanese lemon chicken livers on a pile of rocket leaves	Piece of smoked mackerel + German potato salad + 2 bought cooked beetroots, chopped
Remember at each meal: Sit down, slow down, chew properly				

Resources and recommended suppliers

The Gut Makeover favourite foods

Almond milks

Almond milk without nasties – Provamel unsweetened
http://provamel.com/uk/products/almond-drinks/
almond-unsweetened

Ecomil sugar-free almond milk
www.ecomil.com/en/sin-lactosa-sans-lactose-dairy-free/
ecomil-almond-milk-sugar-free-bio-1-l/

Organic kefirs and other fermented milks

Bio-tiful do a great organic kefir, and also a Russian drink called Riazhenka
http://biotifuldairy.com
Bio-tiful is available for delivery by Ocado
www.ocado.com/webshop/product/Biotiful-Dairy-
Organic-Kefir/247798011

Nourish kefir
www.nourishkefir.co.uk
Nourish kefir is available for delivery by Abel & Cole
www.abelandcole.co.uk/kefir-organic-nourish-250ml

Coconut kefir (good option for dairy-sensitive individuals who can't tolerate fermented milk kefir)

Rhythm
www.rhythmhealth.co.uk/shop/?gclid=CM6B75_-
v8sCFfQW0wod_xkIDA

Fermented miso

Clearspring (they have several, but this particular one would be *Gut Makeover*-friendly because it is unpasteurised). The soya and rice in it is fermented, and although these are to be avoided in the rest of the diet, I suggest trying them specifically here, as many individuals find they can digest them in miso because they have been fermented. www.clearspring.co.uk/collections/traditional-japanese-miso/products/organic-japanese-brown-rice-miso-paste-unpasteurised

Gluten-free baking powder

Doves Farm
www.dovesfarm.co.uk/flour-and-ingredients/baking-powder-1-x-110g/

Pressure cooker

I use a pressure cooker made by Fissler (www.fissler. co.uk) which I find safe and reliable. It has two saucepans; a deep one for big stews and curries, and a shallow one, which is handy for making smaller batches of food. It also has a step you can put inside the deep saucepan for steaming potatoes (useful if you want to cook in batches, cool down and store in the fridge to create prebiotic resistant starch for your gut).

Sauerkraut (unpasteurised, live)

Morgiel
http://morgielfoods.co.uk
www.planetorganic.com/morgiel-sauerkraut-270g-21944/21944/

Raw Health
www.rawhealth.uk.com/product-562-7.html

Thai curry paste

A gluten-free red curry paste with no additives or preservatives
www.thaitaste.co.uk/products/view/curries-for-all-tastes-pastes-kits-sauces/red-curry-paste-gang-ped

Supermarkets

At the time of writing, Tesco, Sainsbury's and Asda are all supplying Eastern European brands of kefir.

Ocado currently supplies the organic kefir by Biotiful mentioned on p. 196, but it is still not available in Waitrose at the time of writing.

Aldi and Lidl supply their own mixes of linseeds/flaxseeds cheaply, and are good places to go to stock up on nuts and seeds cheaply.

Tesco and Sainsbury's both stock frozen black cherries, which taste sensational and are a welcome change from frozen blueberries. I usually fill a drawer of my freezer with them if making a visit to Tesco.

References

Alang, N. and Kelly, C. (2015). 'Weight gain after fecal microbiota transplantation.' *Infectious Diseases Society of America*. (2), 1.

Beirão, et al. (2014). Review article: 'Does the change on gastrointestinal tract microbiome affect host?' *The Brazilian Journal of Infectious Diseases*. 18. (6). 660–663.

Bischoff, et al. (2014). 'Intestinal permeability – a new target for disease prevention and therapy.' *BMC Gastroenterology*. 14.189.

Blaser, M. (2015). 'The microbiome revolution.' *The Journal of Clinical Investigation*. 124. 10.

Brown, K., et al. (2012). 'Diet-induced dysbiosis of the intestinal microbiota and the effects on immunity and disease.' *Nutrients*. 4. (8). 1095–1119.

Byrne, C., et al. (2015). 'The role of short chain fatty acids in appetite regulation and energy homeostasis.' *International Journal of Obesity*. 1–8.

Campbell, A. (2014). Review article: 'Autoimmunity and the gut.' *Autoimmune Diseases*. doi.org/10.1155/2014/152428

Cassidy, A., et al. (2015). 'Higher dietary anthocyanin and flavonol intakes are associated with anti-inflammatory effects in a population of US adults.' *American Journal of Clinical Nutrition*. 102. (1). 172–81.

Cho, I., et al. (2012). 'Antibiotics in early life alter the murine colonic microbiome and adiposity.' *Nature*. 488. (7413). 621–6.

Chowdhury, R., Warnakula, S., Kunutsor, S., Crowe, F., Ward, H., Johnson, L., Franco, O., Butterworth, A., Forouhi, N., Thompson, S., Khaw, K., Mozaffarian, D., Danesh, J., Angelantonio, E. (2014). 'Association of dietary, circulating, and supplement fatty acids with coronary risk: a systematic review and meta-analysis.' *Ann Intern Med*. doi: 10.7326/M13-1788

Clemente, et al. (2012). 'The impact of the gut microbiota on human health: an integrative view.' *Cell*. 148.

Crous-Bou, M., et al. (2014). 'Mediterranean diet and telomere length in Nurses' Health Study: population based cohort study.' *BMJ*. doi: http://dx.doi.org/10.1136/bmj.g6674

Daskalaki, D., et al. (2009). 'Evaluation of phenolic compounds degradation in virgin olive oil during storage and heating.' *Journal of Food and Nutrition Research*. 48.1. 31–41.

De Felippo, C, et al. (2010). 'Impact of diet in shaping gut microbiota revealed by a comparative study in children from Europe and rural Africa.' *PNAS*. 107. 33.

De Souza, R., et al. (2015). 'Intake of saturated and trans unsaturated fatty acids and risk of all cause mortality, cardiovascular disease, and type 2 diabetes: systematic review and meta-analysis of observational studies.' *BMJ*. doi: http://dx.doi.org/10.1136/bmj.h3978

My Drink Aware (2015). https://www.drinkaware.co.uk

Estruch, R., et al. (PREDIMED Study Investigators) (2013). 'Primary prevention of cardiovascular disease with a Mediterranean Diet.' *The New England Journal of Medicine*. 368:1279–1290.

Farrell, R., and Kelly, C., (2002). Review article: 'Celiac sprue.' *The New England Journal of Medicine*. 346. 3.

Fasano, A. (2011). 'Leaky gut and autoimmune diseases.' *Clinic Rev Allerg Immunol*. doi: 10.1007/s12016-011-8291-x.

Flint, H. (2012). 'The impact of nutrition on the human microbiome.' *Nutrition Reviews*. 70. S10-S13.

Flint, H. and Scott, K. (2012). 'The role of the gut microbiota in nutrition and health.' *Nature*. 9. 577–589.

Graham, C., Mullen, A., Whelen, K. (2015). 'Obesity

and the gastrointestinal microbiota: a review of associations and mechanisms.' *Nutrition Reviews*. doi: http://dx.doi.org/10.1093/nutrit/nuv004

Guarner, F. (2015). Review article: 'The Gut Microbiome: What do we know?' *Clinical Liver Disease*. 5. 4.

Haenen, D., Zhang, J., Souza da Silva, C., Bosch, G., van der Meer, I., Arkel, J., van den Borne, J., Gutierrez, O., Smidt, H., Kemp, B., Müller, M., Hooiveld, G. (2013). 'A diet high in resistant starch modulates microbiota composition, SCFA concentrations, and gene expression in pig intestine.' *The Journal of Nutrition*. doi: 10.3945/jn.112.16967

Hale, L., Chichlowski, M., Trinh, C., Greer, P. (2010). 'Dietary supplementation with fresh pineapple juice decreases inflammation and colonic neoplasia in IL-10-deficient mice with colitis.' *Inflammatory Bowel Diseases*. doi: 10.1002/ibd.21320

Hao, Q., et al. (2011). 'Probiotics for preventing acute upper respiratory tract infections.' *Cochrane Review*. doi: 10.1002/14651858.CD006895.pub2

Hanief Sofi, M., et al. (2014). 'pH of drinking water influences the composition of gut microbiome and type I diabetes incidence.' *Diabetes*. 63. 632–644.

Harcombe, Z., et al. (2015). 'Evidence from randomized controlled trials did not support the introduction of dietary fat guidelines in 1977 and 1983: a systematic review and meta-analysis.' *BMJ Open Heart*. doi: 10.1136/openhrt-2014-000196

Higgins, J. (2014). 'Resistant starch and energy balance:

impact on weight loss and maintenance.' *Critical Reviews in Food Science and Nutrition*. 54. 9.

Hulston, C., et al. (2015). 'Probiotic supplementation prevents high-fat, overfeeding-induced insulin resistance in human subjects.' *British Journal of Nutrition*. 113. 596–602.

Human Microbiome Project Consortium (2012). 'Structure, function and diversity of the healthy human microbiome.' *Nature*. 186. 207–214.

Jones, D.S. and Quinn, S. (eds) (2005). *Textbook of Functional Medicine*. WA: Gig Harbour.

Johnson, D. (2013). 'Fecal transplantation for C *difficile*: A How-To Guide.' http://www.medscape.com/viewarticle/779307

Kaplan, J., et al. (2015). 'The emerging field of nutritional mental health: inflammation, the microbiome, oxidative stress, and mitochondrial function.' *Clinical Psychological Science*. 1–17.

Keenan, M., et al (2015). 'Role of resistant starch in improving gut health, adiposity, and insulin resistance.' *American Society for Nutrition*. 6. 198–205.

Khoruts, A. et al. (2010). 'Changes in the composition of the human fecal microbiome after bacteriotherapy for recurrent Clostridium difficile-associated diarrhea.' *Journal of Clinical Gastroenterology*. 44. 354–360.

Kumura, H., et al. (2004). 'Screening of dairy yeast strains for probiotic applications.' *American Dairy Science Association*. 87. 4050–4056.

Le Chatelier, E., et al. (2013). 'Richness of human

gut microbiome correlates with metabolic markers.'
Nature. 500. 541–546.

Leach, J. (2013). Interviewed by Chris Kresser. *Revolution Health Radio Show.* 'You are what your bacteria eat: the importance of feeding your microbiome – with Jeff Leach.' November 20.

Leeman, M., Östman, E., Björck, I. (2005). 'Vinegar dressing and cold storage of potatoes lowers postprandial glycaemic and insulinaemic responses in healthy subjects.' *European Journal of Clinical Nutrition.* 59, 1266–1271.

Lepage, et al. (2012). 'A metagenomic insight into our gut's microbiome.' *Gut.* doi: 10.1136/gutjnl-2011-301805

Malhotra, A. (2013). 'Saturated fat is not the major issue.' *BMJ.* doi: http://dx.doi.org/10.1136/bmj.f6340

Malhotra, A., DiNicolantonio, J., Capewell, S., (2015). Editorial: 'It is time to stop counting calories, and time instead to promote dietary changes that substantially and rapidly reduce cardiovascular morbidity and mortality.' *BMJ Open Heart.* doi: 10.1136/openhrt-2015-000273

Marieb, E., and Hoehn, K. (2007). *Human Anatomy & Physiology.* 7th ed. Pearson: San Francisco.

Marild, K., et al. (2012). 'Pregnancy outcome and risk of celiac disease in offspring: A nationwide case-control study.' *Gastroenterology.* 142. 1. 29–45.

Moreira, A., et al. (2012). Review article: 'Influence of a high-fat diet on gut microbiota, intestinal permeability and metabolic endotoxaemia.' *British Journal of Nutrition.* 108. 801–809.

NHS Choices (2015). Doctors call for change to alcohol advice. www.nhs.uk/news/2011/10October/Pages/alcohol-advice-royal-college-physicians.aspx

Nobel, Y., et al. (2015). 'Metabolic and metagenomic outcomes from early-life pulsed antibiotic treatment.' *Nature Communications*. 6. 7486.

Obregon-Tito, A. (2015). 'Subsistence strategies in traditional societies distinguish gut microbiomes.' *Nature Communications*. doi: 10.1038/ncomms7505

Oyebode, O., et al. (2014). 'Fruit and vegetable consumption and all-cause, cancer and CVD mortality: analysis of Health Survey for England data.' *Journal of Epidemiol Community Health*. doi: 10.1136/jech-2013-203500

Perez-Jiminez., et al. (2010) 'Identification of the 100 richest dietary sources of polyphenols: an application of the Phenol Explorer database.' *European Journal of Clinical Nutrition*. 64. 112–120.

Petyaev, I. and Bashmakov, Y. (2012). 'Could cheese be the missing piece in the French paradox puzzle?' *Medical Hypotheses*. http://dx.doi.org/10.1016/j.mehy.2012.08.018

Rostami, K. (2012). 'A patient's journey: Non-coeliac gluten sensitivity.' *BMJ*. doi: http://dx.doi.org/10.1136/bmj.e7982

Santos, C., et al. (2013). Review article: 'Effect of cooking on olive oil quality attributes.' *Food Research International*. http://dx.doi.org/10.1016/j.foodres.2013.04.014

Sapone, A., et al. (2012). 'Spectrum of gluten-related

disorders: consensus on new nomenclature and classification.' *BMC Medicine*. 10. 13.

Shen, W., et al. (2014). 'Influence of dietary fat on intestinal microbes, inflammation, barrier function and metabolic outcomes.' *Journal of Nutritional Biochemistry*. 25. 270–280.

Shreiner, A., Kao, J., Young, V. (2015). 'The gut microbiome in health and in disease.' *Current Opinion in Gastroenterology*. 31 (1). 69–75.

Simopoulos, A. (2001). 'The Mediterranean diets: what is so special about the diet of Greece? The scientific evidence.' *The Journal of Nutrition*. 131. 11.

Smith, R. (2014). 'Are some diets mass murder?' *BMJ*. doi: http://dx.doi.org/10.1136/bmj.g7654

Smyth, A., et al. (2015). 'Alcohol consumption and cardiovascular disease, cancer, injury, admission to hospital, and mortality: a prospective cohort study.' *The Lancet*. doi: http://dx.doi.org/10.1016/S0140-6736(15)00235-4

Sofi, F., et al. (2013). Review article: 'Mediterranean diet and health.' *Biofactors*. 39. (4). 335–42.

Suez, J., et al. (2014). 'Artificial sweeteners induce glucose intolerance by altering the gut microbiota.' *Nature*. doi: 10.1038/nature13793.

Sun, J. (2014). Commentary. 'Artificial sweeteners are not sweet to the gut microbiome.' *Genes & Diseases*. 1. 130. 131.

Tanaka, T. and Shimazaki, K. (2005). 'Screening of dairy yeast strains for probiotic application.' *Journal of Dairy Science*. 87. 12.

Teixeira, T., et al. (2012). 'Potential mechanisms for the emerging link between obesity and increased intestinal permeability.' *Nutrition Research*. 32. 637–647.

Tillisch, K., et al. (2013). 'Consumption of fermented milk product with probiotic modulates brain activity.' *Gastroenterology*. 144. 7. 1394–401.

Ursell, L., et al. (2012). 'The interpersonal and intra-personal diversity of human-associated microbiota in key body sites.' *Journal of Allergy and Clinical Immunology*. 129.(5).1204–8

Van Nood, E., et al. (2013). 'Duodenal infusion of donor faeces for recurrent Clostridium difficile.' *New England Journal of Medicine*. 368. 407–415.

Van Nood, E., et al. (2014). 'Fecal microbiota transplant-ation facts and controversies.' *Current Opinion in Gastroenterology*. 30. 1. 34–39.

Vassallo, G., et al. (2015). Review article: 'Alcohol and gut microbiota. The possible role of gut microbiota modula-tion in the treatment of alcoholic liver disease.' *Ailment Pharmacol. Ther.* 41 (10). 917–927.

Velasco, J. and Dobarganes, C. (2002). 'Oxidative stabil-ity of virgin olive oil.' *European Journal of Lipid Science*. 104. 661–676.

Velasquez-Manoff, M. (2015). 'Gut microbiome. The peace-keepers.' *Nature*. 518. 11.

Volta, U. (2014). 'Gluten-free diet in the management of patients with irritable bowel syndrome, fibromyal-gia and lymphocytic enteritis.' *Arthritis Research & Therapy*. 16. 505.

Walker, A., et al. (2010). 'Dominant and diet-responsive groups of bacteria within the human colonic microbiota.' *The ISME Journal.* 5. 220 230.

Yang, Y., et al. (2005). 'Long-term proton pump inhibitor therapy and risk of hip fracture.' *JAMA.* 296. 24. 2947–2953.

Zarrinpar, A., et al. (2014). 'Diets and feeding pattern affect the diurnal dynamics of the gut microbiome.' *Cell Metabolism.* 20. 1006–1017.

Index

Acknowledgements

Firstly, thank you to my husband Markus and my children Hanna and Max for keeping me sane during the writing of this book, and for being there for me while I was so busy working on it. Big hugs to you all. A big thank you to the Guided *Gut Makeover* group: Tamsin, Natalie, Caroline, Imke, Celia, Martina, Fee, Amy, and Lynn, with whom I was working with during this period. I learn so much from you, my clients. Thank you Jane Sturrock, my top-class editor, for suggesting this book and for being such a big supporter of *The Gut Makeover* approach, which she and colleagues have followed – with successful results! Thank you Hannah Robinson, Charlotte Fry and Jeska Lyons for all your help along the way and for getting the gut message out there. Thank you Jon Elek, my agent, for making this book happen. Thank you Charlotte Fraser, PR and nutrition supremo, for all your support and belief.